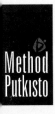

Method Putkisto

Stretch yourself slim in 30 days

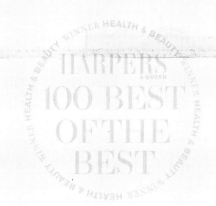

THE BODY
LEAN
&LIFTED

Marja Putkisto

First published 2003 by
A & C Black Publishers Ltd.
37 Soho Square, London W1D 3QZ
www.acblack.com

ISBN 07136 6653 6

Note: Whilst every effort has been made to ensure that the content of this
book is technically accurate and as sound as possible, neither the author nor
the publishers can accept responsibility for any injury or loss sustained as a
result of use of this material.

Text and cover design by Jocelyn Lucas
Photography director: Marja Putkisto
Photography on page viii, xi, 4, 6 © Kaj Ewart
Cover and inside photography © Jukka Asikainen, Studio Helander, Helsinki
Illustrations © James Wakelin
Models: Ulla Mannila, Hanna Laiho

Make-up by Outi Hautamaki; clothing supplied by Piruetti

A & C Black uses paper produced with elemental chlorine-free pulp, harvested
from managed sustainable forests.

Printed and bound in Singapore by Tien Wah Press (Pte) Ltd.

Method Putkisto can only be taught by qualified and authorised instructors.

I dedicate this book to my loving husband Francis Mitchell. Thank you for your ability to acknowledge when it is time to move on in life! Also to my wonderful Mitchell family.

CONTENTS

Acknowledgements vi

Foreword ix

Preface xi

Introduction 01

THE BASICS 03

The Principles behind Method Putkisto 05

Set your personal targets 10

Different types of stretching 13

The five elements of Method Putkisto 20

Your first two days 23

Consolidation 43

Before you begin 47

Questionnaire 52

THE METHOD PUTKISTO 4 WEEK PROGRAMME 55-122

week one: LEARNING THE FUNDAMENTALS 56

week two: WORKING TOWARDS A DEEPER, LONGER STRETCH 57

week three: LONG, INTENSIVE STRETCHING 58

week four: DECISIONS AND CONSOLIDATION 59

THE STRETCHES 60

Stretch and Stabilising banks 123

Elements affecting your results 135

How to measure the results 139

Results questionnaire 142

Moving on! 144

ACKNOWLEDGEMENTS

Thank you to everyone involved in producing this book. Special thanks to Newby Hands, Health and Beauty Director at Harpers & Queen Magazine, for her acknowledgement and vision, and also Lucia Ferrari. Thank you to Harpers and Queen Magazine for their nomination to the '100 best' list.

Sue Carpenter for her ability to reach through her writing 'straight to British people's hearts.' Also thanks to Karen Ewerett and Paivi Ylanen Martin.

Sonia Wilson for her trust and courage, Charlotte Jenkins, Hannah McEwen, Rosanna Bortoli and Jocelyn Lucas from A&C Black Publishers for being such an enjoyable and supportive team to work with.

Jukka Asikainen and Marjanne Helander for your exquisite skill, and also Kaj Ewart. Photographer Kari Hakli for teaching me how photos enable you to catch a special moment. Minna Huovinen for all your hard work. Reetta Ronkko for your great professionalism. Models Ulla Mannila (my friend and very first Method Putkisto client 18 years ago, now a mother of two) and Hanna Laiho for your beautiful modelling. Also Sandy Hullet and Tony Culver for their professionalism and support.

Special thanks to the Finnish Cultural Foundation for their award to Method Putkisto. The Method Putkisto Institute Finland and UK Management team: Jarmo Ahonen, Pirjo Nevalainen, Francis Mitchell, Martin Christie, Minna Ekblom and Kelly Hathaway. To all Method Putkisto instructors and instructor trainees for your trust and dedication.

All my faithful clients over the years, especially Levana and Morris Marshall, Beatrice von Silva Tarouca Larsen and Lisa Spiro. Also thanks to Aida, Avril, Lucy, Anthony and all my faithful Method Putkisto studio clients.

I would also like to thank the following people who have offered their support during an important time in my life, and who have influenced my thoughts during the writing of this book. Paula Day, Vicky Stace, Anoushka

Method Putkisto instructor training, workshops and sessions:

METHOD PUKISTO INSTITUTE
56 Derby Road
London
SW14 7DP
Tel. 020 8878 7384
www.methodputkisto.com

The Method Putkisto video *The Body Lean & Lifted* follows the programme introduced in this book, and can be ordered using the contact details above.

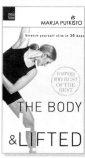

Boone, Dominique Jansen, Shan Williams and Gordon Thomson. Thank you to the UK organisations who were open-minded and trusting towards my work; Steven Purdew from Health Farms UK and Andrew and Mary Lee from Tapestry Holidays. Thank you to the Millennium Dance 2000 team – Donald McLennan, Ikky Maas and Jacqui Mitchell for being forward thinking and allowing us to have the time and support to work with your dancers. Thanks to the Dancers' Development Fund and Riccardo Mariti for your vision and for helping Method Putkisto to get into the right people's hands.

Finally to all my friends and the valuable people who have shown their loyalty over the years. Thank you!

To order the small balls as featured in some of the exercises, please send a cheque payable to 'Method Putkisto Ltd' at the following address:

Method Putkisto Institute
56 Derby Road
London
SW14 7DP

Balls cost £23 each plus p&p (exact postage amounts are detailed on the website **www.methodputkisto.com**).
For queries, please email **smallprops@methodputkisto.com**

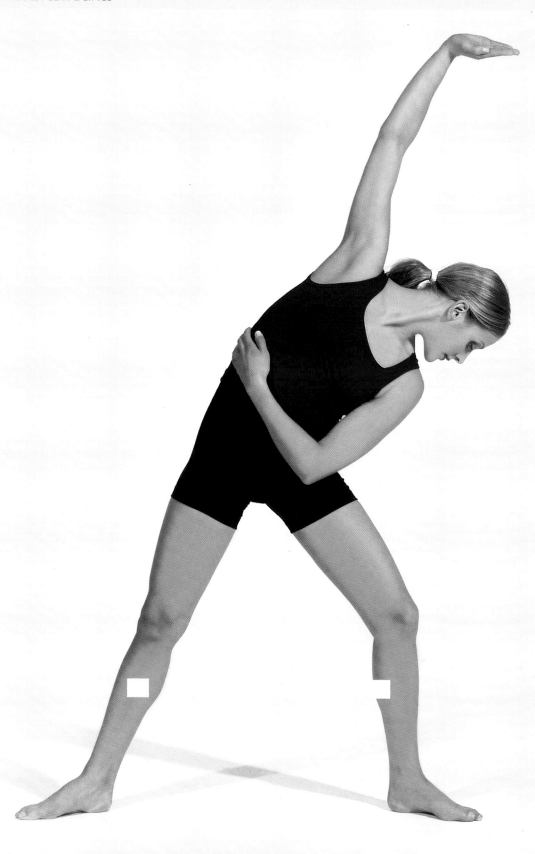

FOREWORD

It has been my privilege to know Marja Putkisto and her unique way of changing the body. In a world where people suffer from various problems with their joints and muscles, Method Putkisto teaches the benefits of a more balanced posture, better flexibility and improved muscular function and control.

I studied physiotherapy in America, before graduating from the School of Nursing and Rehabilitation in Helsinki. I have worked as a team physiotherapist in 10 World and European Championships, and 4 Olympic Games (from Seoul in 1988 through to Sydney in 2000). Throughout this time I also worked as the physiotherapist for the Finnish National Ballet Company.

I have had one of the best seats in the house to observe developments in sport and dance over the last 25 years. I realised that very few people knew how to work on their muscular balance, and it made me really appreciate this method in improving joint and muscle health.

There are a number of different types of exercise that will improve your mind-body connection and muscular balance. However, Method Putkisto is unique for the ease with which you can change your body using central control, breathing, stretching and flexibility. The method is precise in character, gentle for the body, and extremely efficient. It will change your posture, muscular balance and the way you use your body.

Modern society poses increasing health problems, as more people lead relatively sedentary lifestyles, with static desk jobs. It is easy to understand why so many people suffer from joint and muscle problems, with their bodies so tight, unfamiliar and full of 'blind spots' that they find no real pleasure in physical activity.

For these reasons, I wholeheartedly recommend Method Putkisto to you, regardless of your exercise background or medical history. I am sure you will enjoy the exercises, and the results.

Jarmo Ahonen
Educational Director, Method Putkisto Institute
Physiotherapist, Finnish Olympic Teams & Finnish National Ballet Company

"I firmly believe that there is no limit to how much you can improve your body and its potential. I am so grateful that I followed my intuition at a time when I was not able to identify the problems and sensations that I felt. I had a constant awareness my body was not in the right place."

PREFACE

I have now been teaching Method Putkisto for 19 years and Pilates for 12 years, and throughout this time more weight has been given to my original theories. **Muscle length has a profound effect on the position and movement of our bodies.** It is such a simple, visible fact – yet still so difficult to grasp.

Over the last 20 years I have taught numerous clients from very different backgrounds, and I truly believe that no one should have to suffer with aches and pains or discomfort due to lack of flexibility and shortened muscles. Saying 'I'm not very flexible,' 'I'm not able to touch my toes,' or 'my stomach will never be flat,' is the same as saying 'my muscles are so *tight* that I am unable to do this'.

It is only now that I am fully able to understand the effects of an operation I had in my early childhood, because my hip was underdeveloped and needed correction. My legs were held in a static 90-degree position for a number of months, after which my parents were told that the problem had been corrected and my hip sockets had developed normally. Although this was true to a certain extent, I had already got into the habit of holding my body in a particular position, and as a result my muscles became imbalanced during my growing years. The initial problem had only been solved on a superficial level and I grew up 'off-centre'. Although I looked healthy on the outside, I felt restricted on the inside.

Many years later, I began to feel that the muscles on one side of my body were getting tighter. I was very keen on ballet and never missed a lesson. However, despite my dedication and concentration, there were movements that felt impossible to master. Every time I practised pirouettes, I always seemed to find myself at a different end of the classroom compared with the rest of the group! I kept trying, but always experienced the same problem. I felt increasingly disappointed and frustrated.

All of a sudden I was struck by the theory that the cause of the problem was that the whole of my body was too short on the inside. The feeling was so strong that I started accumulating the knowledge needed to create a more complete picture of what was happening to me. I realised that the solution to overcoming the imbalance was simply to stretch my shortened muscles to a length that would allow my pelvis to fall in its neutral position, which allowed my body to move freely. This was the beginning of the Method Putkisto deep-stretching programme.

The change in my body has been far greater than I could ever have dreamt. I can now say with certainty that I have transformed my entire body – I don't think there is a single bone in the same position! The position of my ribcage has improved, I have a reformed waistline, my hips are realigned and my legs are straighter. While lengthening the muscles around my neck I was able to find the correct resting position for my head. When I finally mastered my breathing technique I found that my metabolism improved, my lymph flow became more efficient, and I lost the puffiness and bloating caused by water retention. I have been lucky enough to witness similar changes taking place in a great number of my clients. The best advertisement for this Method really is the visible results.

I concentrated on developing Method Putkisto as aerobics reached a peak in the early 1980s. While the rest of the fitness world was celebrating the music, the beat and the ability to 'feel the burn', I felt that I was working in another universe! However, I persevered with the programme and continued to work on it with my small but dedicated client base at the National Opera and Sibelius Academy in Finland.

I concentrated on perfecting the long, intense, precise stretches and mastering the breathing technique. It was quite an extraordinary feeling when suddenly the world around me started to calm down. Finally, often disillusioned, people began looking around for a less traumatic, less energetic form of exercise. The time for Method Putkisto had arrived.

The Method Putkisto Institute has now been training professional instructors since 1996. The opportunity to train talented people has been a great privilege and it's fantastic to see how my instructors and their clients are enjoying success with the Method.

Method Putkisto works on a 'back to basics' approach, and slots in happily alongside other established methods such as Pilates and Yoga. When you lengthen the tight muscles of your body with precision, your enjoyment of these other disciplines will increase as you find yourself able to execute positions with ease.

It is my great pleasure to introduce you to Method Putkisto. Work hard, and remember, if there are short muscles preventing you from moving, stretch them! Listen to your body and maintain your sense of humour – it will be well worth it. Welcome to the programme and enjoy…

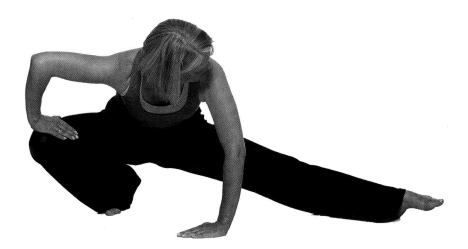

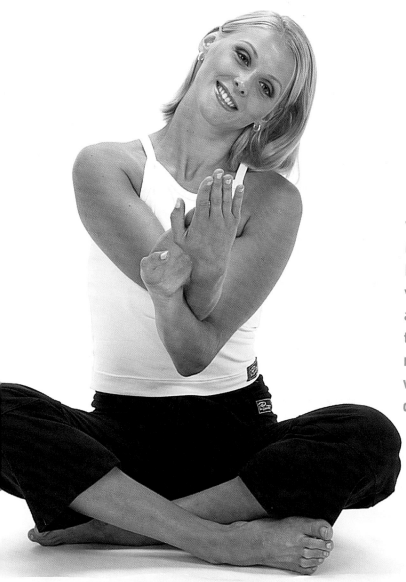

For a healthy life and a beautiful body!

The Method Putkisto programme offers a way forward for anyone wishing to improve their long-term health, well-being and looks. Method Putkisto starts with the very basics, by looking at the activities that you do every day – the way you breathe, walk, sit, run, turn and twist. In other words, the way you use your body during each day of your life.

INTRODUCTION

Following Method Putkisto results in toned, flexible, healthy muscles and a well supported posture. You will find you have a lifted waistline, an opened chest and shoulder line, a realigned pelvis, strong, healthy legs and reduced cellulite. Mastering the breathing technique will result in increased energy levels. The Method alleviates back pain and maintains strong, healthy bones. Best of all, you can learn all of this on your own, by following the clear, concise explanations given during the programme. The aim of Method Putkisto is to improve your health and well-being forever.

WHO IS METHOD PUTKISTO SUITABLE FOR?

The Method is suitable for people of any age and of all fitness levels, from those who spend a lot of time sitting in offices to professional sports people, singers, actors and performers. It is particularly relevant to people with modern-day problems – people who want to reach a greater understanding of the problems affecting their bodies on a daily basis.

Method Putkisto complements other body techniques and therapies, and can be followed on its own or in conjunction with other forms of exercise.

> *Method Putkisto is one of the most sensible, effective and body-changing (if not potentially life changing) methods of exercise I have tried.*
>
> NEWBY HANDS, HARPERS & QUEEN

1

> *Method Putkisto is essentially a method of stretching.... but it cannot be compared to the post-workout stretches with which most of us are familiar. That would be like comparing a marathon runner to someone doing a two-mile fun run.*
>
> **Newby Hands, Harpers & Queen**

THE BASICS

How to use this book

You may be eager to get started and therefore tempted to skip some sections in order to start on the stretches straight away. However, it is vital that you take time to sit down and learn the fundamentals of Method Putkisto. 'The Basics' section that forms the first part of this book will teach you a new approach and language for reshaping your body. Please make sure you understand this vital part of the programme before you embark on the deep stretches.

Following the programme will provide mental and physical 'breathing space' for your body, and maintaining the results is much easier and less demanding than the programme itself. In fact, it is the most satisfying part for most Method Putkisto enthusiasts.

The programme does require hard work and commitment. You may be a working mum, a company director, or you may be retired. You may be tied up with hundreds of everyday tasks and not able to fully focus at this moment in time. Be realistic about the time you can spend on the programme and understand that even following the exercises in a lighter way will substantially improve your health and well-being, although it will take a bit longer to achieve the same results.

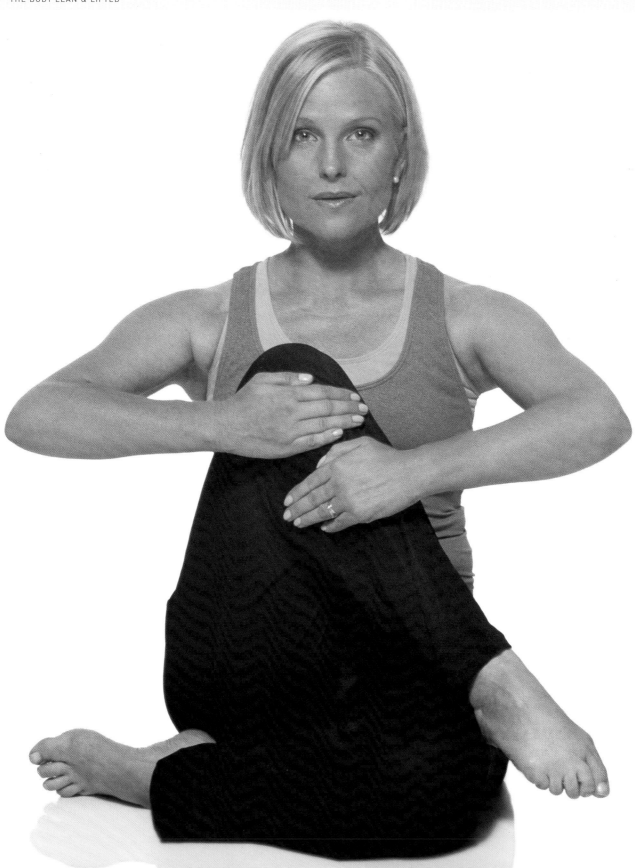

The principles behind
METHOD PUTKISTO

In principle, each muscle should be longer than the bones it supports, or the moves it initiates. Think of the consequences if your muscles are too short and tight.

We all desire a supple, strong and balanced body. Wouldn't it be nice to have a strong pelvis supporting your waistline, an open shoulder line and good overall circulation as well as high energy levels?

Method Putkisto highlights the consequences of short, tight muscles. Muscle shortness is one of the primary causes of health problems and often prevents people from getting the best results in their chosen sport. Most fatigue, stress and imbalances in the body are due to short, tight muscles, poor posture and inefficient breathing.

Since many of us tend to sit for hours each day, over time our muscles get shorter and tighter, often staying in these shortened positions year after year. The shortened muscles eventually force the body out of alignment and, assisted by gravity, pull us towards the ground. The shoulders roll forwards causing the ribcage to sink closer to the pelvis and hips, resulting in the belly popping out.

This effect becomes visible as a loss of a defined waistline and poor abdominal support. If your muscles are too short and tight around the waist area, it is difficult to achieve beneficial results from any exercise programme, no matter how hard you may work. Eventually, just maintaining a good upright position, which ideally shouldn't require any effort, can become difficult.

THE MOVING BODY

Muscles support our bones, and when muscles contract, our bones move. If your muscles become tight and shortened your bones move closer to each other, holding your body in a restricted position. The efficiency of your body is decreased. Your muscles start working against you instead of working for you – instead of supporting your posture, they end up preventing you from moving freely.

For example, if your hamstrings are tight then they will pull your bottom down, which rotates the pelvis into a tilted position, leading to lower back and pelvic problems. It may also lead to a decreased stride length (during running, for example). As a result tight muscles are often a major factor in sports injuries. If your pectoral muscles are tight around the chest, your shoulders will be pulled forwards, decreasing the ability of the chest to expand, limiting movement of the diaphragm and restricting your oxygen intake.

To solve all these problems, Method Putkisto offers you a programme that includes the following three components:

ONE

Lengthens tight and short muscles

These may be preventing your body from moving freely, or restricting your body from falling into an ideal position. By using the Method Putkisto technique, you will take your muscles into a deeper stretch – beyond the normal stretching you might ordinarily do.

TWO

Strengthens the primary postural muscles of your body

This includes the muscles that are responsible for creating a strong, functional 'core' for your body. Improving these core muscles will help you to achieve better and longer lasting results from the stretching.

THREE

Improves your breathing technique

By learning how to use your diaphragm as the primary breathing muscle, you can bring your body into a position of perfect alignment (or find your 'Centreline' see page 28). The waistline is then lifted and supported by using your diaphragm as an 'inner breathing pump', taking the ribcage away from the pelvis. Following the correct breathing technique supports the stretches by making them more

MUSCLE STRUCTURES AND FASCIAS

Each muscle is surrounded with a layer of *fascia*. Deep within the muscles them-selves you have other *fascias*, which surround smaller structures in the muscle. When you elongate a muscle, you are lengthening the outer *fascia* as well as the deeper *fascias*.

When *fascias* are stretched, the resistance in the muscles eases, the muscles become relaxed and they are able to function more efficiently. The muscles now have space to breathe, and this is one rea-son why it starts feeling good to stretch – the *fascias* become able to glide com-fortably past each other.

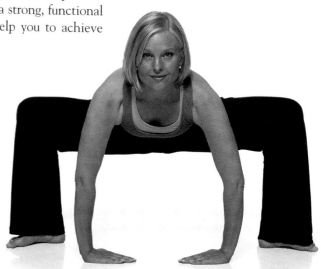

comfortable, and far more efficient. Although within the programme we will work on all three aspects, the primary focus is on mobilising and elongating short muscles.

THE THINKING BODY

In order for you to work on your tight muscles, you need to connect your mind as well as your body. Focus on one muscle group at a time, while maintaining an awareness of your body as a whole. You will learn to use your 'Centreline' (see page 28) as a reference point, as well as techniques that will allow you to focus precisely, and at a deep level. The programme will teach you a new language in relation to your body – a language that you can draw on during your everyday life, whenever you need it.

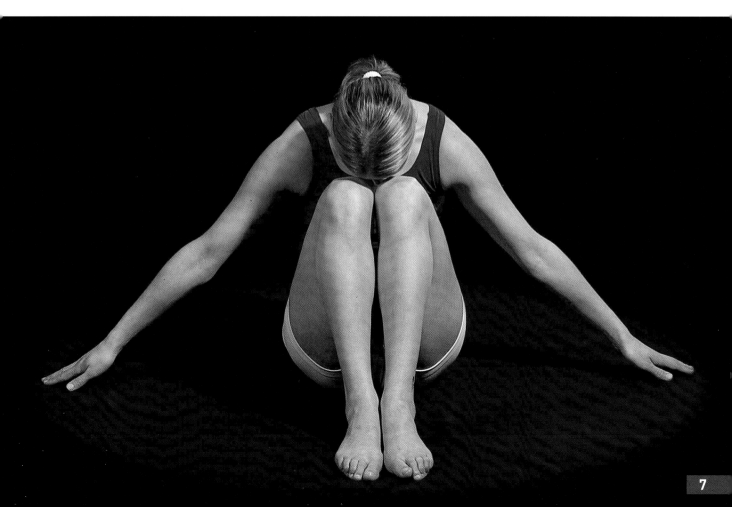

WHAT WILL I ACHIEVE?

The Method Putkisto programme reduces muscle tension and relaxes and strengthens muscles. You can see and feel improvements in your body in 3–4 weeks as it becomes capable of working at a fuller capacity. You can also alleviate long-standing postural problems, pain and discomfort.

Method Putkisto systematically lengthens the primary postural muscles, hamstrings, deep buttock muscles, hip flexors, inner thighs, the muscles around your waist area and your upper body (the diaphragm, chest and upper back muscles).

In an ideal posture, the pelvis should fall naturally into a neutral position and the ribcage should be lifted, relaxed and supported, allowing you to breathe efficiently. An increase in oxygen intake will lead to increased levels of performance that can be sustained over longer periods, and you will soon notice improvements in your energy levels. Improving your breathing technique will also help your body to eliminate toxins and reduce cellulite. Overall, your body 'wakes up' and the muscles function more efficiently. Even your skin colour and facial features will improve.

In response to the deep stretching exercises, your muscles will become stronger. The number of *sarcomeres* (the building blocks of muscle) inside the muscle cells will increase. When the muscle is permanently lengthened the number of *sarcomeres* will permanently increase – the results are long lasting. You will get stronger through stretching!

The most noticeable benefit of the programme is the change to your body shape – you will be leaner, and your posture will be lifted!

THE METHOD PUTKISTO PROCESS

1 Develop an efficient breathing technique
2 Lengthen short, tight muscles (deep stretching)
3 Identify and strengthen the primary postural muscles
4 Get to know your own body
5 Apply the new skills to your everyday life and physical activities.

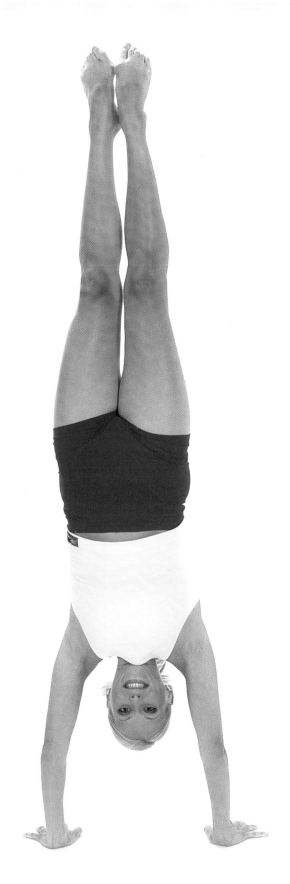

Set your
PERSONAL TARGETS

We all have our own individual fitness targets and needs, relating to our lifestyle and age. As you get to know your body better, you will be able to identify exactly what you feel is essential for its healthy development. Before you embark on the 4 week Method Putkisto programme, ask yourself the following questions. They will help to bring some important issues relating to your body to the forefront of your mind!

WHAT IS YOUR PHYSICAL HISTORY?

- How has your muscular balance developed over the years? Perhaps you have not focused or worked on your body for a long time. Think about the reasons for this.
- Have you ever suffered from any serious illnesses, injuries or operations that have placed stress on your body?
- Have you ever performed stretches to help you to recover after exercising?

HOW WELL DO YOU KNOW YOUR OWN BODY?

- How aware are you of your own body?
- Have you ever set boundaries or limitations for yourself in terms of your physical performance; 'I can't,' or 'I'm not able to?'
- Are you aware of your current physical state in respect of your age, and are you setting your targets too low or too high?

HAVE YOUR PHYSICAL CIRCUMSTANCES CHANGED?

- Are you entering a new period in your life when you need to find a different way of looking after your physical well-being, for example, recovering from a pregnancy or an operation?

- Perhaps your lifestyle is becoming increasingly demanding, and you are looking for a new way to improve your physical well-being?

WHAT CHANGES DO YOU WANT TO MAKE TO YOUR BODY?

Perhaps you are aware of the realistic potential of your body but are not certain how to achieve it. Explore your muscular balance. Think about the position of your body, and how your muscle length and strength can affect it.

- Have your movements become more limited over time?

- Are you able to comfortably maintain your posture?

- Have you paid attention to changes in your posture over recent years? If so, are you aware of the reasons which have lead to this? For example, maybe a change of job has meant that you spend more time sitting in a static position at a desk, or spending more time travelling to and from work.

- Are you aware of tension in your body?

- Are your muscles tight, or are you carrying pain and discomfort in your body?

- Have you followed other exercise programmes in the past, and how did you feel about the results? Did you achieve that flat stomach, or improve the shape of your buttocks, thighs or calves?

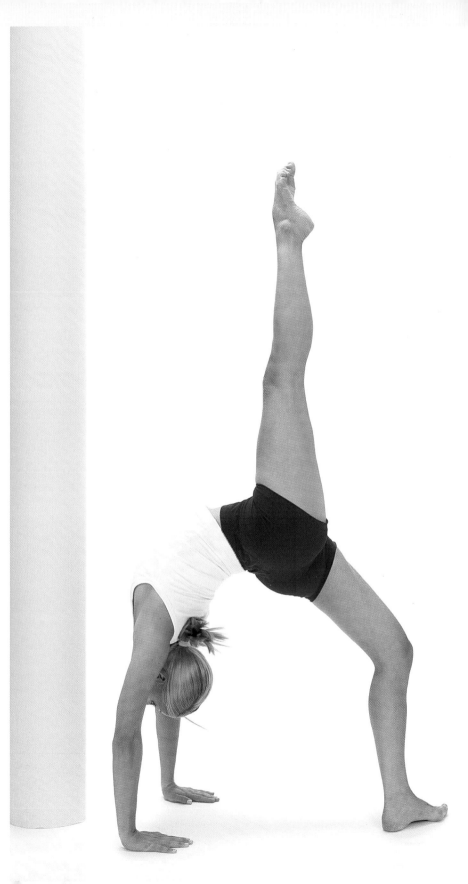

Different types of
STRETCHING

The Method Putkisto programme focuses on stretching the core muscles of your body, so it's important to consider the different types of stretching, and the different types of tissue involved every time you stretch.

1 NORMAL STRETCHING

Before taking a muscle to its new length, you first have to relax it. Only then can you work efficiently on long stretching exercises. In a normal stretch (the type that you may use as a warm-up before working out at the gym or going for a run) the muscle will reach its current full length in around 30 seconds.

2 DEEP STRETCHING

Where a normal stretch ends, a deep stretch begins. A deep stretch will take the muscle to a new length. In order to achieve this you need to visualise the muscle being stretched, and the tension being released. This requires more time than a normal stretch and you will need to work towards a minimum of 2–3 minutes, and as much as 5 minutes for each stretch. As you progress you will learn to work through the natural muscle resistance towards a long lasting, deep muscle stretch.

3 ACTIVE STRETCHING

Active stretching alternates between contracting and releasing the muscle – creating the stretch at the moment of release. The idea is that if you first contract the muscle and then suddenly release it you can catch the muscle unawares and in this split second 'trick' the muscle, elongating it to a new length. It simply has no time to react against sensation of the stretch!

4 PASSIVE STRETCHING

Passive stretching involves applying body weight through a passive muscle, rather than engaging a surrounding muscle to assist the stretch. Body weight gently relaxes the muscle and elongates it. Activity is kept to a minimum in this type of stretching.

ABOUT MUSCLES

OVER-STRETCHING

Muscles are very resilient and it is very difficult for them to be over-stretched when using controlled movement and pressure. They will naturally return to their normal length a little while after a stretch. For this reason it is important to maintain your flexibility throughout your life, and normal stretching is perfectly adequate for this purpose. The difference comes when you begin to work on a muscle which has been in a shortened position for quite some time. This is when you will need to look beyond the normal stretching regime to a deep stretching regime – repeating the programme for several weeks. Muscle damage through over-stretching can sometimes occur in fast sports. However, this usually means that the muscle has been strained or torn, something that won't happen with controlled stretching.

STRETCHING TENDONS

When a muscle contracts small filaments inside the muscle cells move and glide in between each other. If the muscle is contracted when stretched (i.e. if the muscles are cold or tight), then the lengthening of the muscle will take place mainly in the tendon area and other muscular connective tissues, such as fascias.

During very quick, vigorous and uncontrolled stretching the tendon may be damaged – especially if the body is not warmed-up properly. However, well controlled, progressive stretching will improve the elasticity and strength of tendons.

STRETCHING THE LIGAMENTS

Ligaments are found in many joints as part of the joint capsule, and they play an important part in stabilising your joints. Both joint capsules and ligaments are made out of very sturdy connective tissue, including collagen protein. Ligaments

Method Putkisto involves a mix of active and passive stretching. The muscle that you are concentrating on should remain passive, but maintaining your stability and supporting the stretch towards your centre requires controlled activity.

'Good' pain is not something to be afraid of – it means your body is responding normally and you are making progress! It also provides your body with boundaries to work within. You want to avoid the sharp and intolerable 'bad' pain. This is a destructive type of pain that literally does not allow you to stay in a position.

will resist pulling and stretching movements, and it takes time to lengthen them. Quick, repetitive stretching lasting only 7-10 seconds helps the collagen within ligaments to become more flexible and stronger. Often you will see runners performing quick, repetitive stretches at the start of a race for this reason.

However, you need to avoid over stretching the ligaments. If you stretch a ligament for a long period it can become unstable, leading to the joint becoming 'hyper-mobile'. By following the Method Putkisto exercises gently and correctly, and learning the basics – finding your Centreline, Ground Points and Stabilising Points – you will be able to control your joint positions and avoid over-stretching.

STRETCHING NERVES

The Central Nervous System consists of the brain and spinal cord, and smaller nerve channels branch out from between the vertebrae of the spinal cord to the rest of the body. In a healthy functioning body the nerves glide freely through the channels without resisting movement. However, there are areas within the body where the nerves are more susceptible to getting jammed. When this happens they resist movement – especially stretching.

Nerve stretch

The following Nerve stretch is designed to give you an awareness of your nerves and the type of nerve sensation that you must learn to work through.

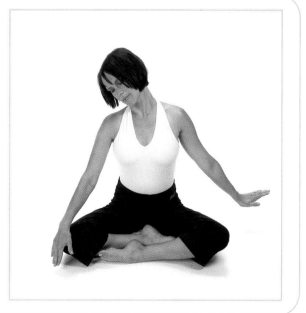

Target to identify the nerves by feeling the sensation they can produce.

Position stand or sit straight. Relax your head to the right, but keep your neck upright. Extend your left arm out at your side. Begin to push the heel of your left hand away from your body, so that your fingers point upwards, and your arm straightens. Gently flex your fingers up and down and feel the nerve 'biting'.

If the movement of a nerve is restricted it **must not be stretched with long lasting stretching exercises**. You will easily recognise if a nerve is jammed when stretching – it will cause an acute, sharp pain, possibly causing a numbness to the toes or fingers. A deep muscle stretch can be likened to a 'sweet pain', whereas nerve pain is more like a 'biting' or 'cutting' pain.

It is likely that you will feel the sensation of a nerve stretch at some point during the exercises, especially as you begin your programme. In the first week you will go through the stretches lightly in order to gently mobilise your body and learn to work through any discomfort that you feel. As you progress, the feeling of nerve stretching will ease, and you will be able to work towards deeper stretches. Don't give up, but continue to work through the programme – it is important to stretch the nerves as long as you are not experiencing the acute, sharp pain described above. At first, concentrate on mobilising your body – easing yourself into the correct stretching position and then releasing, without pushing yourself into a long, deep stretch. Repeating this pattern on each individual stretch will help you to overcome the nerve stretch discomfort, and allow you to work on more effective deep stretches as the month progresses.

STRETCHING THE JOINTS

Between our bones we have joints that differ in size and form. Some have a three-dimensional range of movement (or ROM), for example in the shoulder, and some are almost rigid, for example in the feet, where the bones are closely wedged together.

80% of a joint's stability is dependent on the muscles surrounding that joint. If you force movement in a joint whose natural movement is limited, you may cause irritation in the joint and its surrounding tissue. By the same token, if you stretch naturally loose joints too much without control you may create a 'hyper-mobile' joint that is prone to becoming arthritic at an early age.

Remember that contortion is not the same as muscle flexibility. Method Putkisto will not teach you how to touch your ears with your toes! People who can manoeuvre themselves into all sorts of funny positions are often putting a strain on their joints rather than their muscles. Concentrate on stretching your muscles – **not** your joints – and you will eventually see how increased muscle length will allow your joints to become more stable.

JOINT CAPSULES

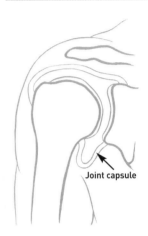

SHOULDER JOINT

Joint capsules surround and support all joints, but there are times when they may also restrict movement severely (for example 'frozen shoulder' where the joint capsule is inflamed and shortened, preventing the sufferer from lifting their arm). While stretching your muscles, you may also cause some stretching to the joint capsules, depending on the joint involved and the position you are holding. Some stretching is inevitable and will cause no harm as long as you concentrate on focusing the stretch on the muscle area.

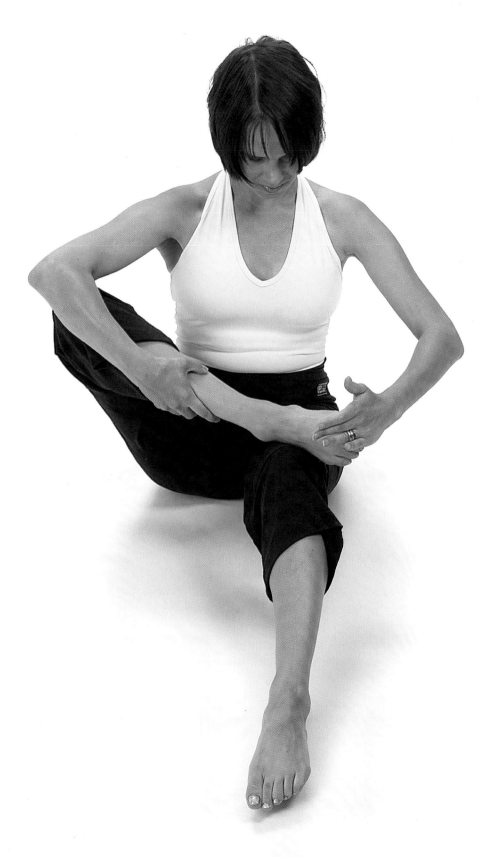

STRETCHING STRONG TISSUE

Some parts of the body are supported by very strong connective tissue structures, providing increased support for areas that will typically be under a lot of stress.

One example is the tissue under the foot that supports the foot arches. Although it is important for tissue in these areas to remain tight in order to function properly, if it becomes too tight then efficient movement can be restricted. Strong tissue needs to be stretched out too.

STRETCHING SCARS

The skin is one large organ – it has many different functions and a great number of nerves pass through it. Skin sensors allow us to feel pressure, temperature changes and even the positions our bodies are in. Normally skin is very flexible and does not resist any movement. However, after accidents, especially burns or large surgical operations, the skin may lose its elasticity due to scarring. It is extremely important that in such cases you start rehabilitation with stretching as soon as possible to reorganise the scarring tissue and to increase its elasticity. Movement is healing, and it is a good idea to explore the idea of mobilising through stretching with your GP or medical adviser.

HOW TO DEEP STRETCH

Compare your muscles to a balloon; it is far harder to get air into the tight neck of a balloon, than into the body of the balloon itself. The same principle applies to muscles. You will easily reach the areas that are loose – it is harder to reach the areas that are tight and not used to movement and circulation. In Method Putkisto, these areas of the body are referred to as 'blind spots'. The body will naturally find its way to the easy, comfortable positions and will resist the difficult areas. Method Putkisto will teach you the skills needed to focus the stretch on a precise area of the muscle. Throughout a stretch it is important to focus on feeling, connecting and understanding your body. This is also part of the process, and will give you far better physical results than forcing or fighting against your body.

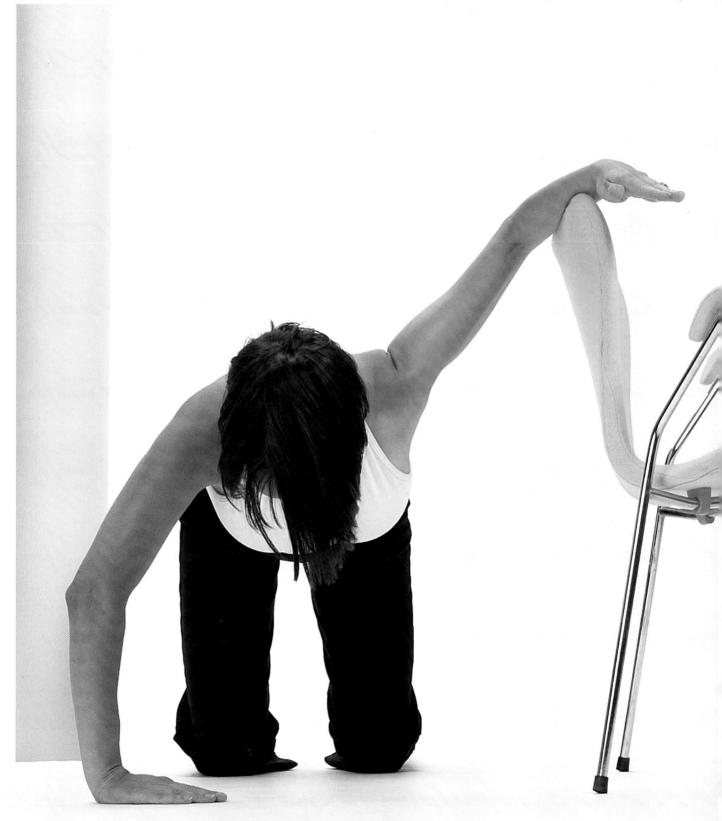

The five elements of
METHOD PUTKISTO

The way you focus, breathe, use space, body weight and time are the elements that create the dynamics required for deep stretching. This builds quality for your movements.

1 FOCUS

Set your target by visualising where the bones and muscles connect. Imagine how it would feel if the muscle was longer and more malleable, or visualise the position that you will achieve at the end of the stretch. Send your muscles a message to relax – work from the inside out, becoming aware of your body. It is necessary to really concentrate in order to feel the stretches in the right area.

Firstly, focus on the parts of your body that are not moving – your Centreline and Stabilising Points (see pages 28–33). Then focus on the area that you want to mobilise. In your mind, isolate the single muscle (or group of muscles) that you wish to lengthen, and focus on them one at a time.

2 BREATHING

Breathing is a vital tool for deep stretching. It creates a rhythmic flow, helping you to time your stretches, as well as contributing to the pressure of your stretches as you inhale and exhale. It also serves to release any discomfort in the stretch. During the programme we use two breathing techniques:

HALF MOON BREATHING
Focusing on the lower lungs (see pages 36–38).

USE YOUR IMAGINATION!

Visualisation is a skill that most of us enjoyed as a child, but one that tends to get neglected in adult life. Remember when you were a child listening to stories, and how you made sense of them in your own mind by creating strong images?

Visualisation in Method Putkisto is exactly same; imagine and visualise how it would feel to have longer, more elastic muscles, and then work towards it. First open your mind to see how you will look and feel, and then go for it!

RISING SUN BREATHING
Focusing on the upper lungs (see pages 36–39).

When you are stretching, focus your breathing on the isolated muscle that you are working on. Imagine the muscle expanding from the pressure created when you inhale. When you exhale, feel pressure easing out of your muscle, creating a flowing sensation.

Following the flow of your breathing as you work on your deep stretching will also help your mind relax. Your muscles will become responsive to the message that you send them, and you will not have to force or push in order to take the muscle to its new length.

3 SPACE

When you stretch a muscle, be aware of the space around you, and of the direction in which you apply and release your body weight. Establish in your mind the part of your body that is moving up, and the part that is moving down. Make yourself aware of the opposite forces that are working to create a stretch.

Stay focused on the target of your stretch – allow your muscles to lengthen until the bones are able to reach the position you want. This spatial awareness will help you in your aim to reach your target position.

4 WEIGHT

To create a deep stretch you need to apply sufficient weight through the muscle using your own body weight. By establishing your Ground Point (see page 26) you can increase, decrease, stabilise and control the amount of weight needed during your stretch. We have a tendency to use too much effort too quickly.

Remember that less is often more – ease and breathe into the stretch, applying body weight gradually. Relax and allow gravity to take over.

Aim to develop an awareness of your body, allowing you to sense when and how much weight you have to apply. Remember, muscles will naturally resist the applied weight. Move and breathe slowly and the muscles will gradually give in, enabling you to elongate them.

5 TIME

The length of time you take on each deep stretch is the key to progress and success.

To reach a deep stretch you need to take more time than with normal stretching. Usually, it requires a minimum of 2 minutes up to 5 minutes. This allows enough time for you to think, feel and work your way through each stretch. However this is a guideline time only. Avoid imposing a rigid time frame when you are deep stretching – especially as you start out on the programme. Instead rely on your own body awareness and common sense.

Deep stretching is a process of focusing, sensing, and feeling over time. Give your muscles time to respond to your message to relax. It will take approximately 5-10 seconds for the electrical impulse sent by your brain to reach your muscle, and for the muscle to respond accordingly by relaxing, allowing you to stretch further. Once your muscle is no longer reacting against the stretch and has become more compliant and passive, continue your stretch until you feel it reach another stage of resistance. Now hang on and keep on focusing on the next step – towards a deeper stretch. Feel the response of your muscles as this will determine the time and action of the stretch – follow the rhythm of your breathing. Above all, relax and take your time!

Note If you recognise the pain of a nerve 'biting' (see page 15) trust your intuition. Allow your body to feel its way through the programme, easing the stretch when you feel you need to.

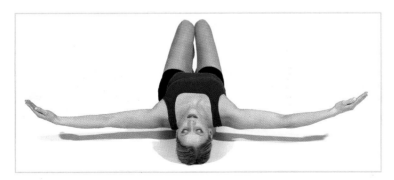

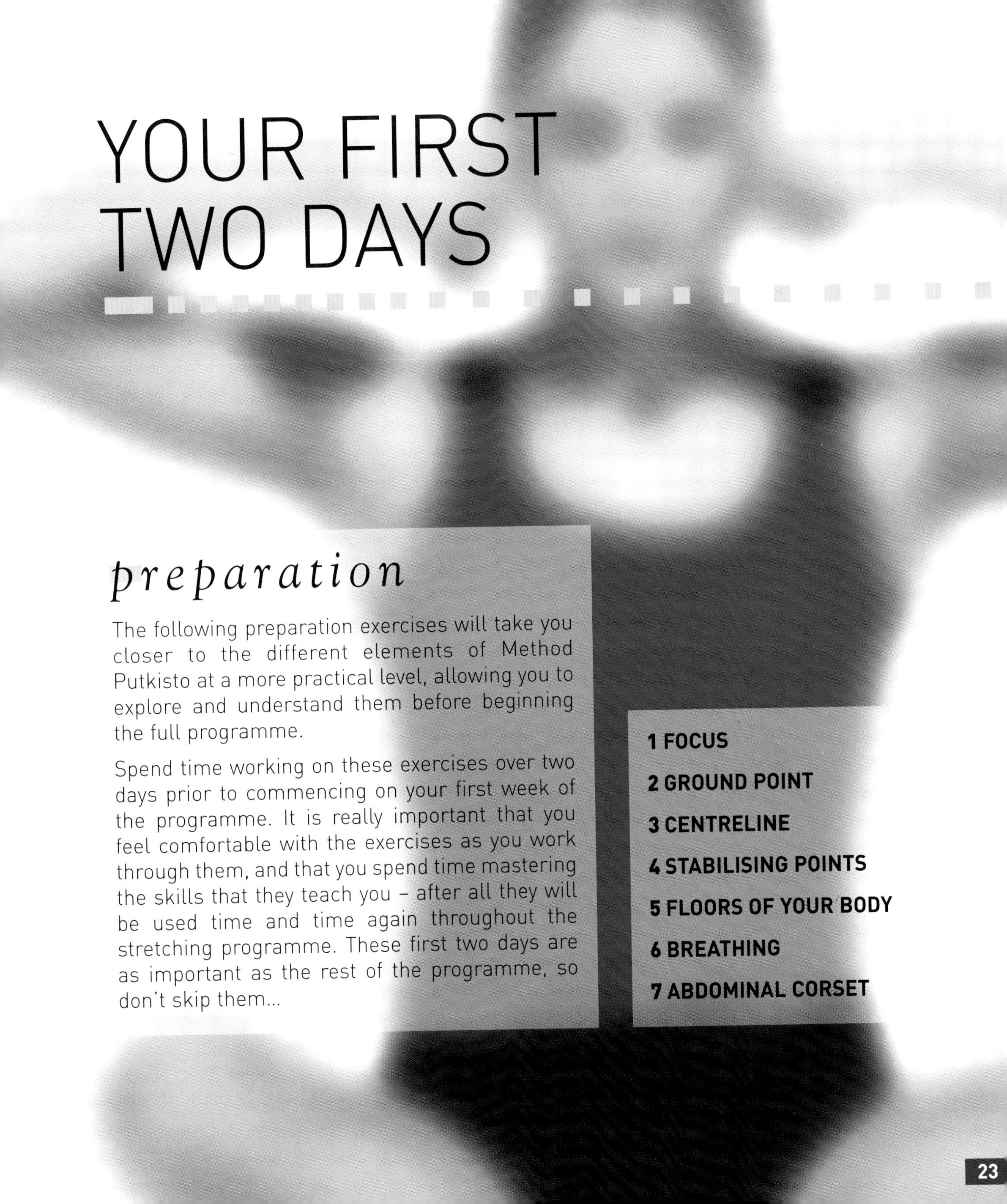

YOUR FIRST
TWO DAYS

preparation

The following preparation exercises will take you closer to the different elements of Method Putkisto at a more practical level, allowing you to explore and understand them before beginning the full programme.

Spend time working on these exercises over two days prior to commencing on your first week of the programme. It is really important that you feel comfortable with the exercises as you work through them, and that you spend time mastering the skills that they teach you – after all they will be used time and time again throughout the stretching programme. These first two days are as important as the rest of the programme, so don't skip them...

1 FOCUS

2 GROUND POINT

3 CENTRELINE

4 STABILISING POINTS

5 FLOORS OF YOUR BODY

6 BREATHING

7 ABDOMINAL CORSET

1 FOCUS

The first important element is the ability to focus your mind. Achieving the correct level of concentration can sometimes seem difficult. As the body's reactions naturally follow the movement of the eye, it is important first to relax your eye muscles, and make sure that your eyes do not wander around. The following two exercises will help you to focus your mind and bring it in tune with your body.

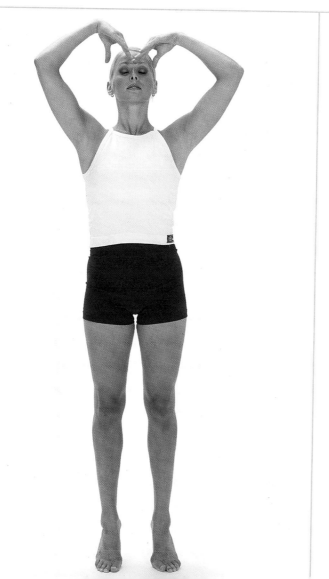

1 FOCUS
Focus point of the eyes

Target to help you to focus; to become aware of the positions of your body.

Position sit upright and place your thumbs on your temples and turn your fingertips to face the tip of your nose. Press your fingertips onto the bridge of your nose at its highest point and press lightly downwards. Relax your eyes and jaw.

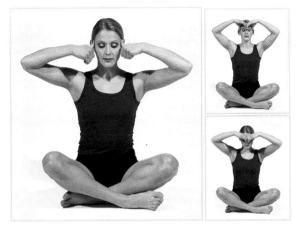

1 FOCUS
Dance of the eyes

Target to relax your eyes, and reach a deeper level of concentration; to find the 'centre' of your eyes.

Position sit upright and place your fingers on the focus point (the same position as described above) and close your eyes.

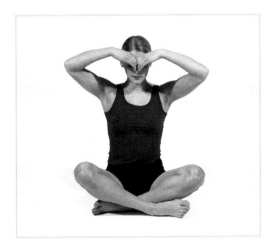

Steps

✳ move your eyes to the upper left corner; return to the centre

✳ move your eyes to the lower right corner; return to the centre

✳ move your eyes to the upper right corner; return to the centre

✳ move your eyes to the lower left corner; return to the centre

2 GROUND POINT

You must learn to use gravity to your own advantage. By bending and extending your arms or legs you can increase, decrease, control and stabilise your stretches by opposing the force of gravity. You can increase the effectiveness of your stretches by using your 'Ground Point' to work against gravity.

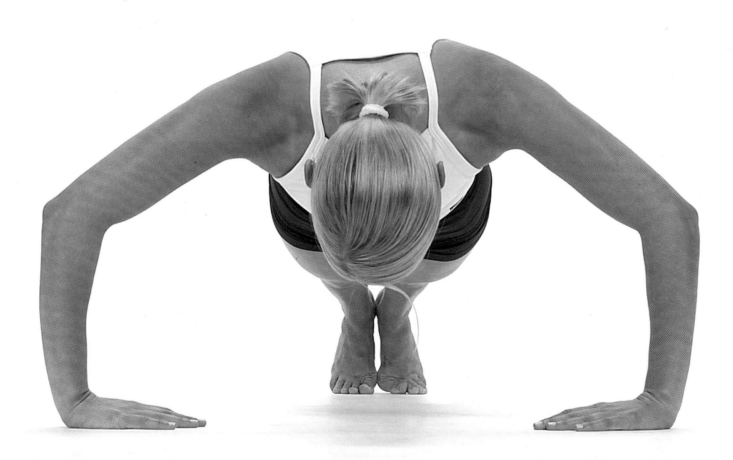

2 GROUND POINT
Find your Ground Point

Position lie on your back, keeping your back straight. Bend your knees and place your heels together, in line with your sitting bones. Press your feet firmly into the ground, observing how your lower back feels lighter.

Release the pressure through your feet, and feel the weight shift back to your lower back. In this way, you are alternating between Ground Points.

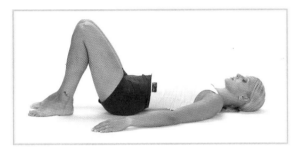

SITTING BONES & TAILBONE

Sitting bones are the bones at the bottom of your spine that take your weight when you sit down. You can locate them by placing your hands under your buttocks and finding the two little bones that protrude downwards. The coccyx is the very lowest part of the spine, and is also referred to as the 'tailbone'. You can turn your tailbone out, or tuck in under – altering the position of your pelvis.

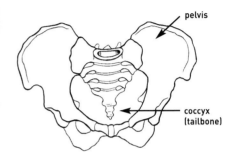

pelvis

coccyx (tailbone)

2 GROUND POINT
Rabbit stretch

Target to find your Ground Point under your hands and feet; to master the use of gravity in your stretches.

Position crouch on the floor and arch your back forwards, bringing your knees towards your chest. Place your hands on the floor and tilt your head down. Relax your body weight towards your heels.

Alternate between shifting your body weight backwards and forwards – first towards your hands and then back towards your feet. Explore the sense of the weight shifting from your feet to your hands and back to your feet again. Keep your knees as close to your chest as possible.

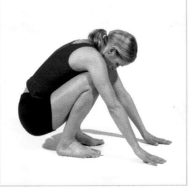

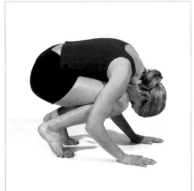

3 CENTRELINE

The 'Centreline' refers to your body's position in relation to gravity. You should be aware of your Centreline in every movement you make. When you are standing up, your Centreline travels vertically in front of the spine from the top of your head to the bottom of your lower back. Working within your Centreline will improve your agility by providing you with a reference point for all your movements, and improving your balance.

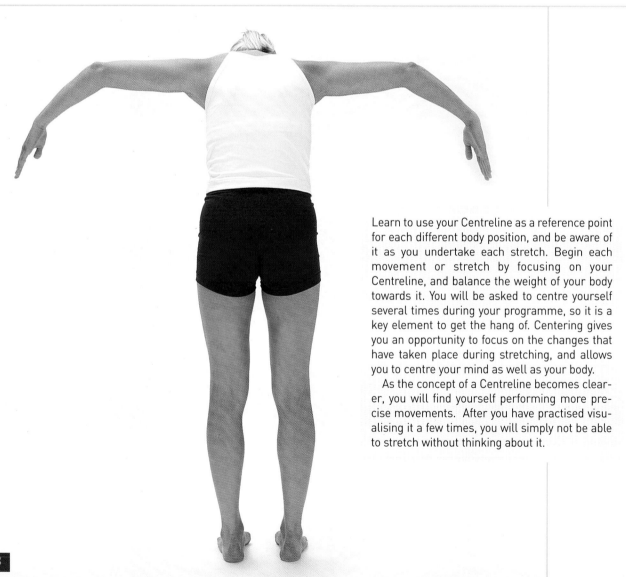

Learn to use your Centreline as a reference point for each different body position, and be aware of it as you undertake each stretch. Begin each movement or stretch by focusing on your Centreline, and balance the weight of your body towards it. You will be asked to centre yourself several times during your programme, so it is a key element to get the hang of. Centering gives you an opportunity to focus on the changes that have taken place during stretching, and allows you to centre your mind as well as your body.

As the concept of a Centreline becomes clearer, you will find yourself performing more precise movements. After you have practised visualising it a few times, you will simply not be able to stretch without thinking about it.

3 CENTRELINE
Travel through your Centreline

Your body weight should always be balanced towards your Centreline, never away from it.

Target to establish your Centreline.

Position lie on your back on the floor, with your knees bent. Place your heels hip width apart, and place your arms flat along the side of your body.

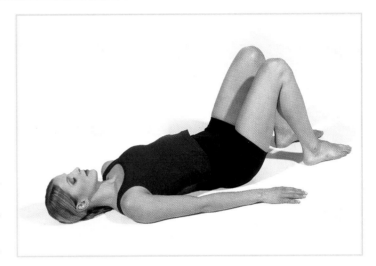

Steps

※ visualise the space within your ribcage – it has a front, sides, and a back. Drop your weight to the bottom of your ribcage. Feel how it falls onto the lowest part. In your mind move your area of focus, visualising your pelvis. Think about the shape of your pelvis from the inside out. The pelvis has sides, a back and is open at the front. It is built in two halves, which are connected to each other through the base of the spine.

※ visualise the two sitting bones. Drop the weight on to the back of your pelvis – towards your sitting bones. In your mind move your area of focus to your spine. The spine begins almost from behind your eye level. From there it continues its way down through your neck to your ribcage, through your ribcage to your waist and pelvis, ending at the tailbone. Your spine has a front, which is at the moment facing towards the ceiling, and a back, which is facing towards the floor. At the front, the vertebrae are rounded. Your Centreline travels in front of the spine – from the top of your head to your tailbone.

※ relax your abdomen and feel the weight on the front of your spine.

※ imagine there is a little man doing somersaults along the front of your spine. Each time a somersault is performed, you can sense the weight of your inner organs dropping onto that part of the spine.

※ turn the tailbone (see page 27) towards your navel, and then away from your navel while visualising your Centreline.

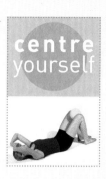

centre yourself

3 CENTRELINE
Centre yourself

During stretching it is important to maintain the sense of your centre and throughout the programme you will be prompted to 'centre yourself' whenever you see the icon above. However, you can repeat the following exercise as many times as you like during your session.

Position lie on your back on the floor with your knees bent, your feet, ankles and knees either together or slightly apart. If you have a little ball or cushion place it between your knees. Place your fingertips on your focus point (see page 25).

Steps

* inhale to prepare

* exhale, pressing your feet firmly into the floor, and then pressing your knees together

* pull up your pelvic floor by 'squeezing' the muscles around your sitting bones

* release the pressure, and repeat the movement again.

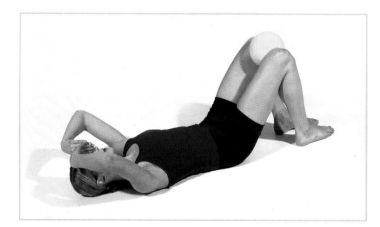

tip
relax as much as possible throughout this movement. This will allow you to feel the deeper muscles activating more easily.

4 STABILISING POINTS

When you perform any movement be aware of the parts of your body that are not moving – these will provide a stabilising force for your body. These stable areas will also provide you with a counter-balance for your stretches.

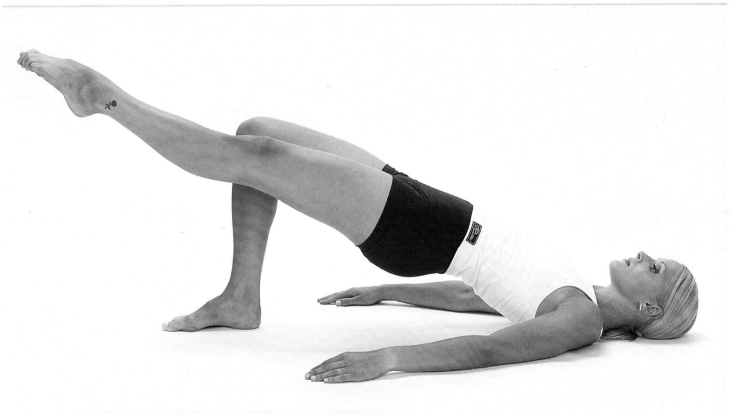

Stabilising Points are internal Ground Points – located within the body and in front of the spine (Centreline), helping you to focus and create very precise movements. Using Stabilising Points you will also be able to maintain contact with your Centreline, find a neutral position for your pelvis, and work more effectively with your abdominal corset and diaphragm.

4 STABILISING POINTS
Find your Stabilising Points
Navel Point

Diaphragm Point

Throat Point

Target to locate your Navel Point.

Position place one of your hands about 3 cm down from your navel towards your tailbone, and in your mind move inwards towards the front of your spine. This is the location of the Navel Point. Working with your Navel Point will help you find a neutral resting position for your pelvis, as you will become more aware of its position during the movements that you make.

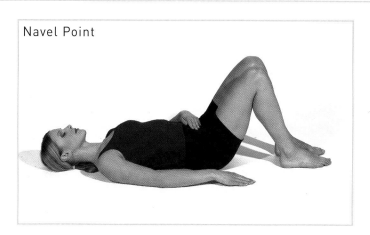

Navel Point

Target to locate your Diaphragm Point.

Position your Diaphragm Point is located around 4-10 cm down from your breastbone towards the middle of your body. Like your Navel Point, it is just in front of your spine. It helps you to control the movement of the diaphragm and Abdominal Corset, and gives you a good reference point when learning any of the movements. It may help to think of the Diaphragm Point as the *central turning point* of your body – it is located at the same place where the spine can move in all directions, allowing you to bend forwards, backwards, sideways and rotate.

The Diaphragm Point is a vital tool for all of the stretches. By holding it towards the front of your spine you will bring your stomach in towards your Centreline. As you breathe imagine the Diaphragm Point moving – it moves down towards your Navel Point as you exhale, and releases upwards as you inhale.

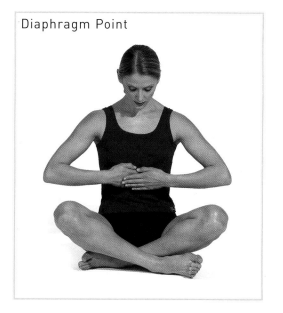

Diaphragm Point

Target to locate your Throat Point.

Position the Throat Point is located at the top of the throat, and is related to the movement of the larynx. When you exhale, the larynx lifts at the same time as the diaphragm.

If you are holding your head out of alignment (tilting it slightly), then the larynx will be unable to move and relax during exhalation. This in turn affects your breathing technique by making it difficult to use efficient diaphragm breathing. By working on the neck stretches further on in the programme, and focusing on your Throat Point, you will be able to concentrate on improving the alignment of your head.

Throat Point

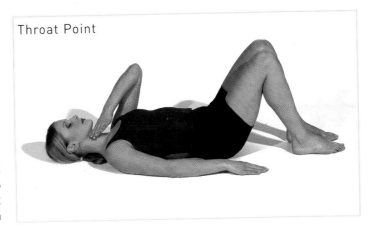

5 FLOORS OF YOUR BODY

There are several horizontal 'floor-like' muscles in your body, such as the pelvic floor and the diaphragm. The pelvic floor consists of a group of muscles located between your tailbone, pubic bone and sitting bones. It forms a strong, elastic, supportive floor for your inner organs.

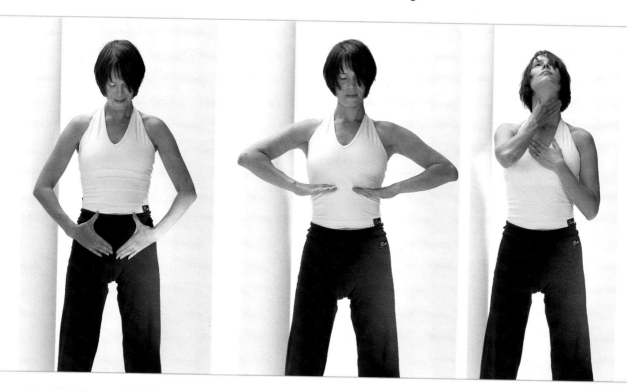

The pelvic floor muscles follow the movement of the diaphragm, moving up and down the Centreline. You will be able to explore this more fully when you connect the floors of your body (in the next exercise) allowing your pelvic floor and diaphragm to work together. By developing support from your Abdominal Corset, you will soon be able to form a functional 'core', supporting your centre and enabling you to control and stabilise all your movements and actions – including breathing – more effectively.

5 FLOORS OF YOUR BODY

Connect the floors of your body

Learn how easy it can be to connect the 'floors' of your body to your Stabilising Points.

Target to locate your First Floor (pelvic floor).

Position lie on your back on the floor with your knees bent; squeeze your knees together, and then squeeze the muscles around your sitting bones.

Steps

* imagine you have string that goes through your body, starting from your tailbone at the back, coming out at your Navel Point at the front. You can pull up your pevic floor by pulling on this string.

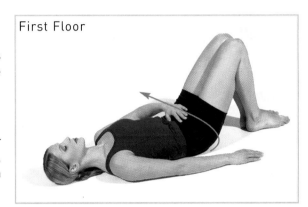

First Floor

Target to connect your First Floor to your Second Floor (diaphragm)

Steps

* pull your Navel Point up towards your Diaphragm. As you inhale, hold your Diaphragm Point down towards your Navel Point.

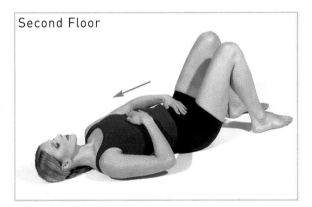

Second Floor

Target to connect with and relax your Third Floor (surrounding your Throat Point)

Steps

* align your head within your Centreline. This will allow you to relax the muscles surrounding your Throat Point when you exhale. It may help to place your hands gently at your throat to help you focus on this movement.

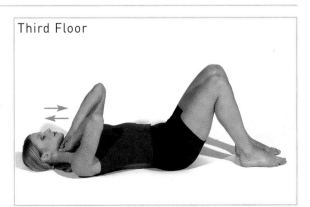

Third Floor

6 BREATHING

Breathing is the true key to power, energy, vitality and life. You breathe to live. Respiration brings oxygen to the blood in order to maintain metabolism and energy production. Breathing out (exhaling) cleanses the body of carbon dioxide so it is beneficial to empty the deepest parts of the lungs where waste gas tends to accumulate.

Finding both my Centreline and the support of my diaphragm has improved my performance in other sports dramatically.

Billy,
Method Putkisto client

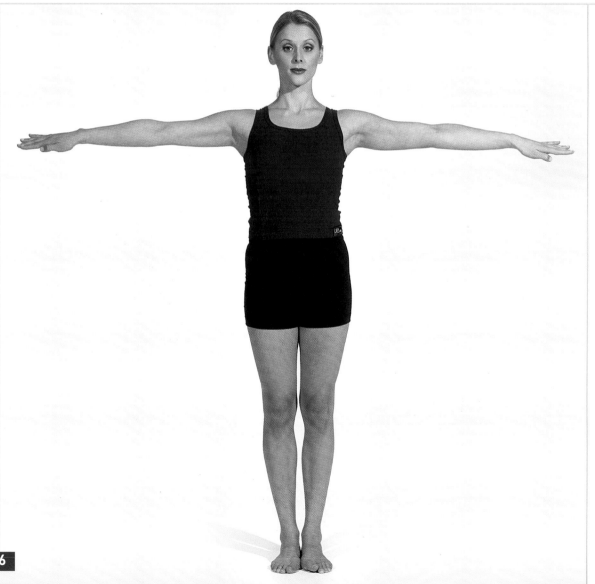

During the programme, one of your targets is to learn how breathing can create a change in pressure within the body, and how you can utilise it like a 'pump' to assist your movement, stretches, posture and voice production.

The breathing exercises on the following pages will help you to understand and connect with your diaphragm to develop an efficient breathing technique. These breathing techniques will be beneficial to you not only in your normal exercise regime, but also in your everyday life.

DIAPHRAGM

The diaphragm is like a floor for your lungs, or a ceiling for your abdominal cavity. Your heart rests on the top of the diaphragm, slightly left of your Centreline. The diaphragm is central to your body and also central to the programme – you can choose to consciously control it just by focusing on its movement, but it will also control itself if you don't. It forms a physical dividing line between the upper and lower body and regulates itself even when you are asleep.

When you inhale, you are actively contracting the diaphragm. Exhalation is passive, with the diaphragm releasing upwards, not requiring any extra effort on your part.

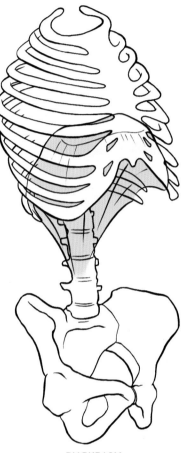

DIAPHRAGM

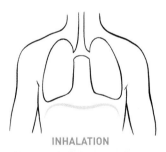

INHALATION

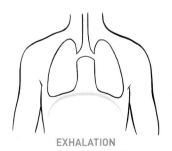

EXHALATION

TAKE A DEEP BREATH

First start with a long exhalation, pause, and then inhale. This will allow you to breathe deeply.

6 BREATHING
Half Moon breathing

Target to learn efficient diaphragm breathing while maintaining a flat stomach, through engaging your Abdominal Corset when breathing in and out; to circulate air to the lowest part of your lungs.

Steps

* imagine your diaphragm within your ribcage, just underneath your lungs. It resembles a parachute in shape and is connected at the sides of your ribcage by your lowest ribs, at the front of the ribcage at the breastbone, and at the front part of your spine just above the pelvis (see diagram on page 37).

* inhale through your nose, and focus on the air reaching the lowest parts of your lungs (your diaphragm will contract during this movement). Exhale through your mouth and feel your diaphragm rising up towards your lungs like a parachute, releasing air as it does.

* squeeze even more air out of your lungs by lightly pulling your abdominal corset towards your Centreline. Use both you abdominal and back muscle to increase your exhalation. PAUSE before the next inhalation.

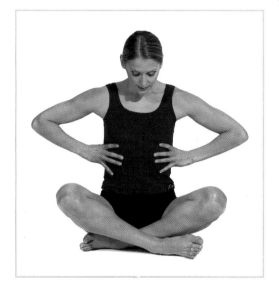

Note The deepest abdominals are like a 'wall'. If you are able to prevent these muscles expanding when inhaling, you will strengthen the abdominal wall. In learning to control your abdominals correctly you will be able to support your inner organs towards your Centreline.

tip

First relax the diaphragm, and don't contract your abdominals until the diaphragm has released up towards your lungs.

6 BREATHING
Rising Sun breathing

Target to become familiar with the upper part of your lungs; to relax the upper chest and muscles around your Throat Point when you exhale.

Position lie on your back on the floor – place a small pillow under your head if it's more comfortable. Put one hand on your chest and the other on the back of your neck. At the back of the neck feel the natural curve inward of the vertebrae (this curve is the same as the inward curve of the lower back). Slightly tilt your chin down, lengthening the back of your neck.

Steps

※ focus on the upper part of your lungs.

※ inhale through your nose, allowing your breastbone to lift gradually as you feel your lungs filling. Limit the downwards movement of the diaphragm, making it very compact. Pause at the end of the inhalation.

※ relax and exhale, allowing your upper chest to expel all the air. Imagine that your ribs are soft and allow yourself to relax further into the outwards flow of air.

※ PAUSE before your next inhalation.

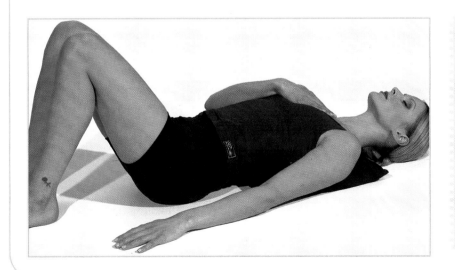

Note If you find it difficult to inhale and exhale deeply, this means that you are either holding too much tension in your upper back, or you are tensing your back muscles without realising it. As you work on your breathing exercises throughout the programme the area between your shoulder blades will eventually expand more as you breathe in.

7 ABDOMINAL CORSET

When stretching, breathing, or performing any movement, it is important to be aware of your Centreline (see p.28). Your abdominal muscles, together with your back muscles, create a corset-like muscle 'band' around your centre; connecting your ribcage and pelvis together and supporting your inner organs towards your Centreline. Throughout the programme you will become more aware of your Abdominal Corset, and working with it will help to improve your every day posture in the long term.

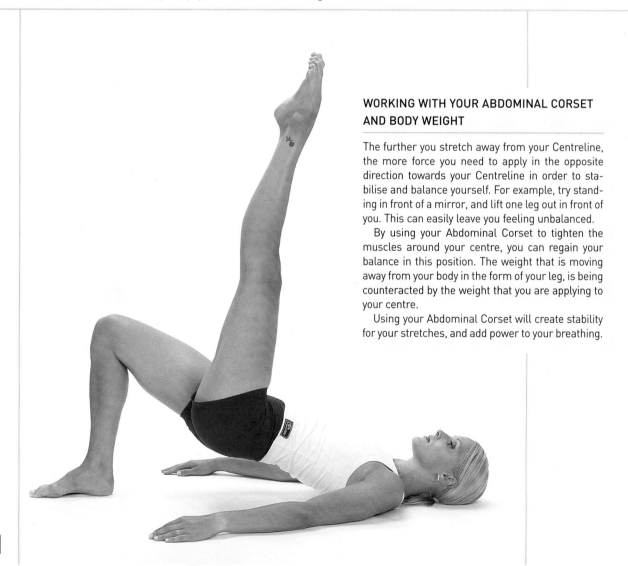

WORKING WITH YOUR ABDOMINAL CORSET AND BODY WEIGHT

The further you stretch away from your Centreline, the more force you need to apply in the opposite direction towards your Centreline in order to stabilise and balance yourself. For example, try standing in front of a mirror, and lift one leg out in front of you. This can easily leave you feeling unbalanced.

By using your Abdominal Corset to tighten the muscles around your centre, you can regain your balance in this position. The weight that is moving away from your body in the form of your leg, is being counteracted by the weight that you are applying to your centre.

Using your Abdominal Corset will create stability for your stretches, and add power to your breathing.

7 ABDOMINAL CORSET
'One ribcage, two arms' principle

Target to locate and work with your Abdominal Corset by using arm movements and Half Moon breathing.

Preparation focus on the Diaphragm Point and use it as a reference point for the next exercise.

Position lie on the floor with your knees bent, keeping your feet firmly on the floor. Place your right arm around your ribcage, with your hand on the lower left side of your ribs. Lift your left arm up towards the ceiling, softly pointing your fingers.

Steps

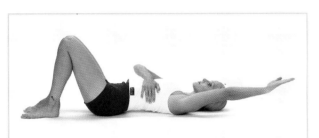

* inhale to prepare.

* begin your exhalation.

* at the end of your exhalation PAUSE, take your left arm over your head and move the shoulder blade of the same arm down to increase the stretch and feel the muscles around your ribcage.

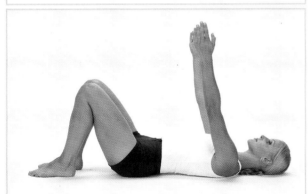

* contract your abdominal muscles towards your Centreline – this will activate your Abdominal Corset.

* as you inhale, imagine that your Diaphragm Point is moving down towards your Centreline at the front of your spine. (This will help you learn to hold your abdominal muscles towards your centre). Use the Diaphragm Point as your Ground Point (really drop your weight onto it and imagine it pressing on your spine). As you exhale, return your arm back to the starting point. Make sure you initiate the movement from your lowest ribs. Don't lift your ribcage or arch your back.

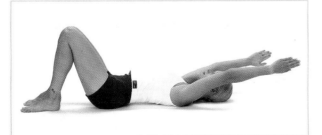

* repeat this movement three times with each arm.

* finally repeat the same movement with both arms three times; taking your arms over your head and returning them to the starting position. Continue to use your Diaphragm Point as your Ground Point.

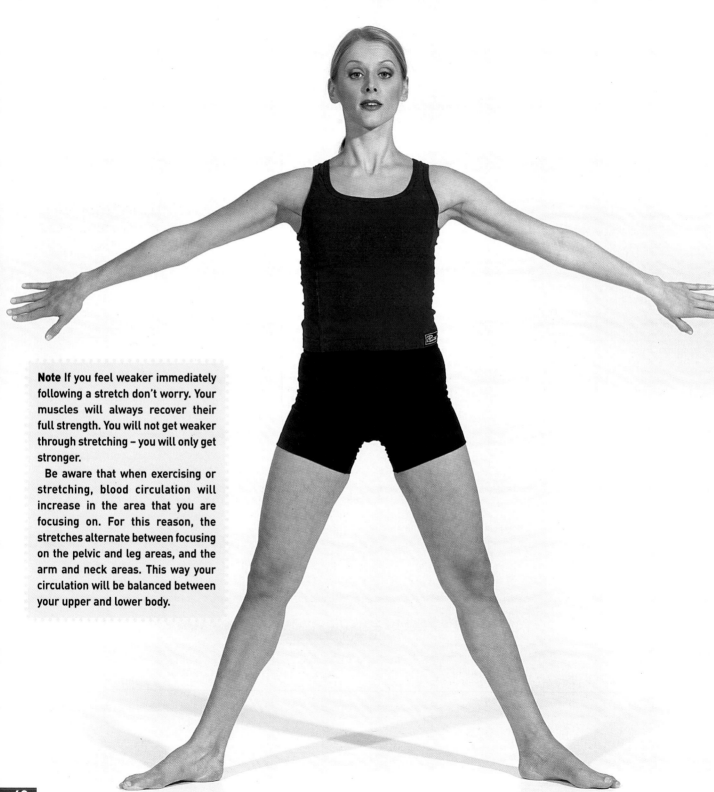

Note If you feel weaker immediately following a stretch don't worry. Your muscles will always recover their full strength. You will not get weaker through stretching – you will only get stronger.

Be aware that when exercising or stretching, blood circulation will increase in the area that you are focusing on. For this reason, the stretches alternate between focusing on the pelvic and leg areas, and the arm and neck areas. This way your circulation will be balanced between your upper and lower body.

CONSOLIDATION

You have now covered the essential elements of Method Putkisto, and at the moment this may seem rather a lot to take in! Now it's important to repeat and master the preparatory work, both physically and mentally. The exercise overleaf is a good way to repeat the basics, combining all the elements.

STRETCHING CHECKLIST

The following checklist will guide you through the main components involved in creating a stretch. The programme teaches you to use the right kind of effort, time and body weight to move your muscles from a normal stretch to deep stretch (see page 13). Imagine that you are now working on one deep stretch (around 3–5 minutes) and visualise the process:

- find the correct starting position, enabling you to drop your body weight onto the muscle.

- establish your Ground Points (see page 26).

- focus on the areas that are not moving – your Centreline and Stabilising Points (see pages 28 & 31)

- focus on the area that is moving – the muscle you are stretching – and visualise its new position.

- use your Ground Points to increase or decrease the weight to through the muscle – stretching the muscle to its full length.

- PAUSE

- use the correct breathing technique stated in each stretch. Concentrate on feeling the pressure increasing and decreasing on the muscle as you inhale and exhale.

- send a message to the muscle to relax and release any discomfort. It will take about 10–20 seconds for the muscle to respond

- now start to take the stretch deeper, until the muscle reaches a new length.

- after the stretch look at yourself in a mirror. You should be able to see the side that you have been stretching is now either higher or visibly more open than the side that you haven't stretched.

Remember:
- the muscle you are lengthening should remain passive, while other parts of your body can be active (Abdominal Corset, Ground Point).

- take your time.

- re-define your Centreline and Stabilising Points.

- after stretching stay warm and avoid heavy exercise; your body needs time to adjust to the new muscle balance.

CONSOLIDATION
Have a ball

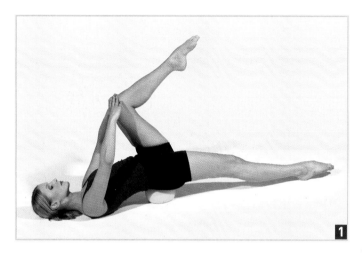

1

Preparation use a small soft ball as shown in the picture. If you don't have one of these it is just as good to use a tightly rolled towel or a small, tight cushion. It needs to be something that will both lift and support your pelvis while you are lying down.

Position lie on your back on the floor with your knees bent, and place your feet on the floor hip-width apart. Press your feet into the floor, and lift your pelvis up into the air. Place the ball underneath your tailbone. Tilt your tailbone, towards your Navel Point.

> **Note** Make sure the ball or towel is not underneath your lower back – it must be underneath your tailbone.

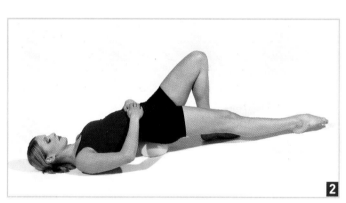

2

Breathing Half Moon

Steps (a)

* relax your eyes and focus on your Centreline.

* inhale using Half Moon breathing (see page 38).

* exhale and relax; move your Navel Point towards your spine. Use your pelvic floor muscles to move your Navel Point closer to your Diaphragm Point.

* lift your left knee towards your chest (picture 1).

* tilt your tailbone further towards your Navel Point.

* relax the Navel Point further towards your

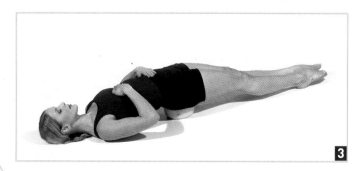

3

*Above all, listen to
your intuition and
common sense!*

spine. Lower your left leg over the ball until your foot is on the floor. This is your Ground Point (picture 2).

✳ focus on relaxing your lower abdominals. Think about the space between the top of your leg and pelvis, and the idea that the bones are moving away from each other.

✳ if comfortable, straighten both your legs out (picture 3). Focus on slowing down your breathing, PAUSE at the end of exhalation.

✳ change legs, repeating the same movement.

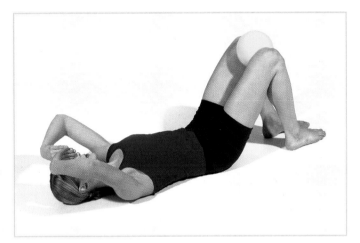

tip

If you feel discomfort, make sure the ball is placed correctly, and that you are not tensing your back.

Steps (b)

 bend both knees, and press your feet firmly on the floor, lift your pelvis off the ball and place the ball or towel between your knees.

✳ place your hands on the 'focus point of the eyes' (see page 25).

✳ roll through your spine. Relax one vertebrae at a time onto the floor, following your Centreline – through your ribcage, waistline and pelvis until your pelvis reaches its neutral position, following the line of the floor (it is not tilted either forward or back). Squeeze the ball, and centre yourself.

Note When your Diaphragm and Navel Point are relaxed towards your spine as you inhale, your body weight is balanced towards your Centreline. If you feel that they are lifting upwards and away from your Centreline, don't worry; the muscles around your waist and back are probably short. As your progress through the programme the weight of your body weight will move closer towards your spine.

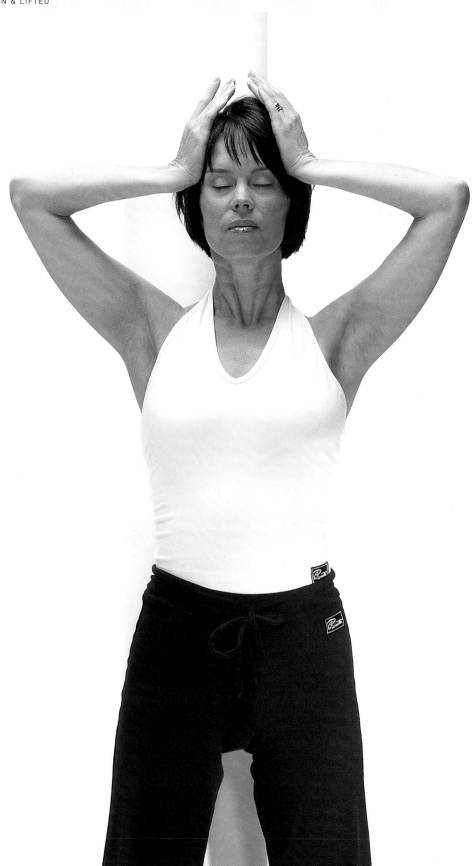

BEFORE YOU BEGIN

THE PRACTICALS

HOW TO FOLLOW THE PROGRAMME

At first go through the programme lightly, to familiarise yourself with the nerve sensations that you will learn to work through. Keep your stretches short and light in the first week. Only after you have done this can you start to build up the intensity of the stretches. Always respect the resting days, as these will give your muscles time to recover and become stronger.

The programme is intensive, but also user-friendly. There will be some days when you will have to go through the whole programme, and other days when you only need to go through the shorter half programme. Be realistic about the time you can spend on the stretches, and how you can fit them in around other commitments. If something unavoidable takes your time and focus away, you can follow the shorter programme as often as you are able to, and start back on the main programme as soon as possible.

WHEN TO FOLLOW THE PROGRAMME

You can choose to follow the programme in many ways. Perhaps you would find it beneficial to divide your session in half, and perform some of the exercises in the morning and some in the evening. If you do choose to follow the programme this way, place the more intensive sessions towards the evening. During your sleep the muscle fibres have time to rest, adjust and re-build, making them stronger.

In the mornings the programme can provide an opportunity for you to wake up and mobilise your body, and you should find the morning session enjoyable

– especially after an intensive evening session. Perhaps you are lucky enough to have the time and space to complete some of the session in your lunch break. It could offer a good way to relax your mind away from work, and leave you feeling refreshed and revived in the afternoon. On the other hand you may find it easier to work on the programme in one go – setting time aside in the evenings and at weekends. Find out what works best for you.

OTHER EXERCISING

After a heavy workout, keep your stretches lighter and likewise avoid doing heavy exercise after a deep stretching session – please don't go to a 'spinning' class straight afterwards! Common sense is a great help with the programme, and you will benefit from your sessions most when you allow your muscles to adjust to their new length through rest, or by combining the programme with light exercises, such as walking. After a long session of stretching your muscles may feel temporarily weaker. However, you will soon recover your normal strength.

If you are a sportsperson and are regularly training and competing then follow the programme out of season – otherwise you may place too many demands on your body.

WHERE TO STRETCH

Never underestimate the effect that the environment and space around you has. Find, or create, a space – it doesn't have to be much more than a large corner – in which you feel relaxed and comfortable. It is good to try and use the same place for all your sessions, as it will help you to concentrate on your programme. Consider the following factors when choosing your environment:

* is there a source of natural light?
* is there good air circulation?
* is the temperature suitable (at least average room temperature – 20°C – with no draught)?
* are there suitable surfaces to support your stretches (a chair or a low table, and sometimes a doorframe)?
* is the environment calming (it may be necessary to take away any clutter)?
* do you have a comfortable floor surface to work on (a mat and cushions)?

Your biggest task is not to go through the programme. It is to create the space, time and peace to allow yourself to concentrate on it!

* do you have the necessary equipment (a small ball or tightly rolled towel, and a band, scarf or belt)?

* are you wearing comfortable clothing that allows you to move freely (always wear something that covers your stomach and lower back to keep your middle warm)?

SAFETY

There is no danger in stretching if you follow the correct technique; always work slowly, paying attention to the various sensations of your body. Your awareness of your own body is what makes stretching safe.

Never stretch inflamed or injured muscles. Be aware of sciatica, lower back, shoulder or knee pain, or any other conditions in these areas. (see 'What is your physical history?' on page 10) If you suffer from any specific medical conditions then you should consult your GP before starting the programme.

HURDLES ON THE WAY

You may find it difficult to feel and sense your body; to get in touch with its 'blind spots' and to work through new movements. At first, the stretches can be uncomfortable and you will experience a certain amount of discomfort. You may find it difficult to relax and focus on the exercise in a way that allows you to increase the movement range of your body in these immobile areas, especially in the lower back, the hips, the top the legs, the neck and the upper back area.

Don't expect to learn everything at once. Method Putkisto is an ongoing process of learning about your body, and as you work through the weeks the elements will become clearer.

COMMITMENT

Trust your intuition but learn to recognise the distinction between not being able to do something and not wanting to do something. We all know that there are a million reasons to say 'I can't,' or 'I'm too busy.' I completely understand that for many people there are a million things to pack into one day. However I strongly encourage you to *make and take the time* for yourself.

You might find it difficult to explain to your friends and family why you have chosen to put aside a month to concentrate on your stretching programme, but the time will pass quickly and the results will be worth it. You may prefer not to talk about what you are doing, keeping it as your own private time. It is entirely your choice. Reward yourself with the knowledge that you are looking after yourself and improving your body. Keep your overall target clear in your mind – to stretch your body to a new shape, to be lean, lifted and pain free. Keep this positive thought in mind and remember that this is a great investment of your time for the future!

If you find it difficult to work on your own, think about getting a small group of friends together. Practising together can be motivating, fun and rewarding.

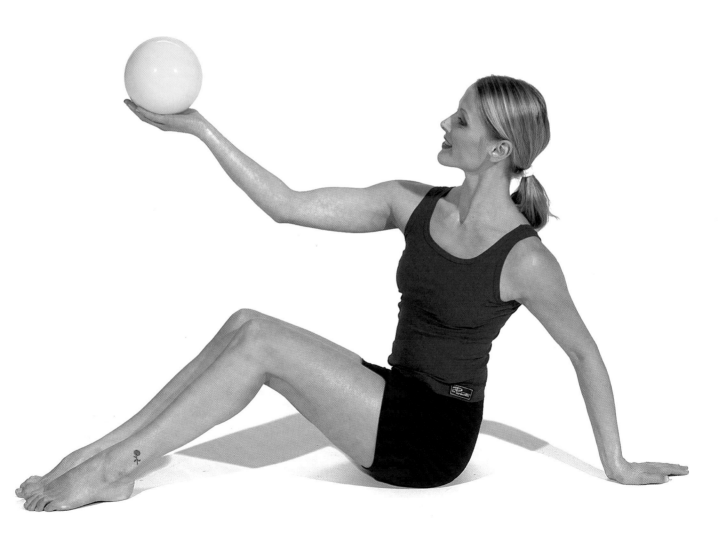

QUESTIONNAIRE

The following questionnaire is for you to answer before you start the programme. Keep a record of your answers, as you will be asked to go through a similar questionnaire at the end. There are no right and wrong answers – the aim is to provide you with some food for thought – allowing you to assess your results with the aid of the final section. You may find that you have a very different physical experience to the one you expected...

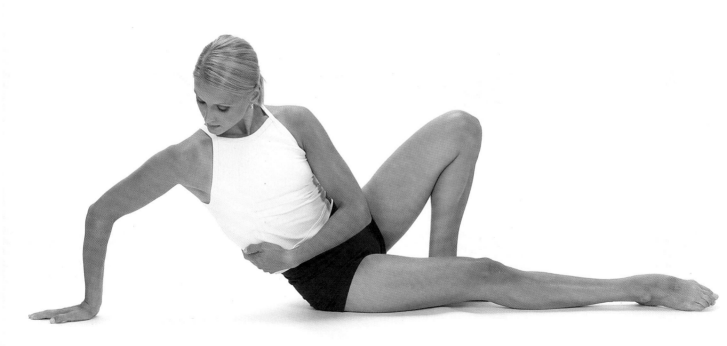

1 How often do you exercise at the moment, and what do you hope to gain from it?

2 What are your expectations of this programme?

3 What kind of improvements would you like to see in your:

appearance?

performance?

4 How would you describe your body? (in three words)

5 How would you describe your posture? (in three words)

6 Rate your energy levels on a scale of 1–4.
(1 = low, 4 = high)

1   2   3   4

7 Rate the quality of sleep you experience on a scale of 1–4. (1 = broken sleep, 4 = well-rested)

1   2   3   4

8 Rate the quality of your breathing on a scale of 1–4.
(1 = shallow, inefficient breathing, 4 = deep, effective breathing)

1   2   3   4

9 Rate your range and ease of movement on a scale of 1-4. (1= difficult movement, 4 = full ease of movement)

1   2   3   4

10 Rate your muscle balance (do you feel shorter or tighter on one side?) on a scale of 1–4.
(1 = severe imbalance, 4 = perfect balance)

1   2   3   4

11 Do your muscles feel elastic or inelastic, on a scale of 1–4. (1 = inelastic, 4 = elastic)

1   2   3   4

12 Rate your flexibility on a scale of 1–4.
(1 = inflexible, 4 = flexible)

1   2   3   4

13 If you feel that you are inflexible, which muscles would you consider to be your primary problem areas?

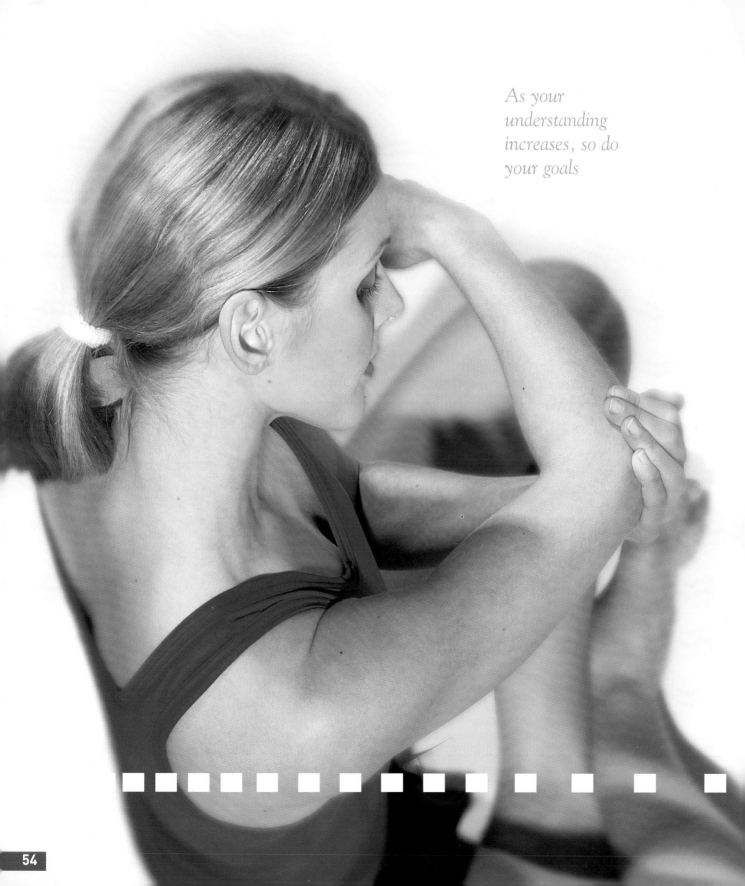

As your
understanding
increases, so do
your goals

THE METHOD PUTKISTO 4WEEK PROGRAMME

Well done! You have already worked hard to learn the essential elements of Method Putkisto, and you are now ready to start on the stretching programme.

The programme itself is simple. There is one stretching programme to follow, and each week you will work on the same stretches, developing an awareness of your body and working towards a deeper stretch. On some days you will be required to work through the whole programme. On other days you will work through a shorter half programme – only working on those stretches marked with a half symbol.

*Feel your
way through*

week one
Learning the fundamentals

✳ **work on the programme 4–5 days a week.**

✳ **go through the full programme 3 times.**

✳ **go through the half programme on 1 or 2 times.**

✳ **keep the stretches short – a maximum of 40 seconds to 1 minute for each stretch.**

✳ go through the programme lightly, concentrating on how you feel and think during each stretch. Spend time exploring the stretches, but do not force or push your body.

✳ focus and mentally connect with the stretches. Getting used to this can at first be as hard as the stretches themselves.

NB You do not have to complete the full programme on 3 consecutive days. You can mix the half programme in-between full programme days and rest days. Find a rhythm that suits you. See the example below.

	Mon	Tues	Weds	Thurs	Fri	Sat	Sun
example a	full	half	rest	full	full	half	rest
example b	rest	full	full	rest	half	rest	full

FOCUS ON THE ELEMENTS

✳ firstly drop your weight, and then transfer it through your Ground Points.

✳ find your Centreline.

✳ establish you Stabilising Points (the throat, diaphragm and navel points.

✳ work on your breathing technique.

✳ familiarise yourself with the nerve sensations that you may feel, keeping the stretches short and light.

✳ get to know your body.

RECOVERY SUGGESTIONS

● drink plenty of water to help cleanse your system

● make sure you rest well in between sessions

● a massage is a good way to release any toxins in your body

Work your way through

week two
Working towards a deeper, longer stretch

* work on the programme 4–5 days a week.
* go through the full programme 3 times
* go through the half programme 1 or 2 times
* work towards holding the stretches for longer – between 1 and 3 minutes

FOCUS ON YOUR PROGRESS

* focus on your Abdominal Corset during this week
* remember to focus first on what is *not* moving (Centreline) and then what *is* moving.

RECOVERY SUGGESTIONS

* drink plenty of water to help cleanse your system
* make sure you rest well in between sessions
* a bath with dead sea salt or essential oils and candles can be a great way to relax

I kept moaning when doing these exercises, but now I can bend over so far that my nose nearly touches my knees!

Kelly,
Method Putkisto client

My shoulder line has opened out and my double chin has disappeared

Lisa,
Method Putkisto client

week three
Long, intensive stretches

*Go for it! This week is not just about doing the programme – it is about the **way** that you do it. This is the main week and you will really feel the difference at the end…*

WEEK OUTLINES

* **work on the programme 5–6 days a week.**
* **go through the full programme 4 times.**
* **go through the half programme 1 or 2 times.**
* **develop the deep stretching method that you have worked towards in the previous week – between 3 and 5 minutes.**

* by week three you will hopefully have become used to dedicating your time and thoughts to the exercises. Remember this week is hard work, but it will provide a real turning point. Just think of the rewards at the end and stay focused!

It's hard to believe but my energy levels are higher than ever before

Francis,
Method Putkisto client

FOCUS ON DEEPENING YOUR STRETCHES

* slow your breathing down.
* spend more time on the breathing exercises to help detoxify your body.
* hold the pause at the end of exhalation.
* focus on working on the deeper layers of your muscles.
* work through the muscle resistance and feel the difference!

RECOVERY SUGGESTIONS

* take time to rest and allow your muscles to rebuild. No intensive exercise classes, long-distance running or weights this week!

Control your
way through

week four
Decisions and consolidation

PREPARE FOR THE LIFE-LONG PROCESS

By the end of the third week you should have reached some conclusions about your progress and your muscular balance. You may also feel that your muscles feel different – more malleable or compliant.

Our bodies are not symmetrical, and they differ in bone structure, shape, size, length and placement. They also differ in muscle length. By now you should have a better understanding of the varying degrees of shortness in your body. Aim to work on the shorter muscles more intensively. If you feel that your pectoral muscles are shorter on the right-hand side of your chest than they are on the left, spend more time working on the shorter side in order to correct the imbalance. Focus not only on the balance between your right and left side, but also the balance between the surface muscles and the deeper muscles. Trust your intuition and make decisions based on how *you* feel.

* **work on the programme 4–5 days a week.**
* **go through the full programme 3 times.**
* **go through the half programme 1 or 2 times.**

DEVELOP YOUR OWN PLAN

Think about the new skills that you have learnt and identify the muscles that you feel need more work. Think about how you can find the time and space to incorporate a stretching programme into your life that meets your personal needs. Be free to create your own programme.

* identify any areas that you feel need more work, and focus your deep stretching programme on these areas.

* allow yourself to make discoveries and change your areas of focus as you see you body in a new light.

* be aware of your body.

* make choices about the life-long process that can lead you to long-term well-being, suppleness and health!

THE STRETCHES

PROGRAMME OUTLINE

WARM-UP

Swimming
Criss-cross & loop half
Centreline pull

CENTERING EXERCISES

Dance of the eyes
Travel through your Centreline
Have a ball

FIND YOUR GROUND POINT

Rabbit stretch
Toe stretch
Triangle stretch

FIND YOUR BREATHING PUMP

Bow stretch on the floor half
Bow stretch

DEEP STRETCHES: LEGS, PELVIS AND BUTTOCKS

Humming bird stretch half
Swan dive
Lizard stretch half

Swan stretch half
Swan rotation
Sitting stork stretch half
Standing stork stretch
Box split stretch

FIND YOUR UPPER LUNGS
Rising Sun breathing

DEEP STRETCHES: CHEST
Butterfly half
Butterfly kneeling
Swallow bird I
Swallow bird II

DEEP STRETCHES: BACK AND NECK
Somersault stretch
Cross-arm neck stretch
Tall crane stretch I
Tall crane stretch II
Swan neck stretch half
Otter stretch half
Sitting bat stretch

WARM-UP

Swimming

Target to warm-up.

Breathing Rising Sun.

Position stand with your feet together or hip width apart – whatever feels more comfortable.

Steps

* inhale using Rising Sun breathing.

* place your hands on your Diaphragm Point area (picture 1).

* exhale, extending your arms out and away from your body, with the back of your hands facing each other.

* inhale, and open your arms to the side of your body (picture 2).

* continue the movement by bringing your arms round to the back of your ribcage and dropping you head (picture 3) – you can slightly arch your upper back.

* focus on your Diaphragm Point.

* run your arms around your ribcage back to your Diaphragm Point.

* lift your head and exhale deeply – expelling the air from the bottom of your lungs. This requires the use of your abdominal corset (see page 40).

* repeat the movement 3–5 times; starting slowly and becoming faster.

Note Use your Abdominal Corset to support your centre

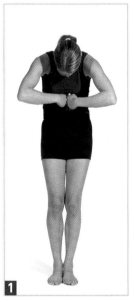
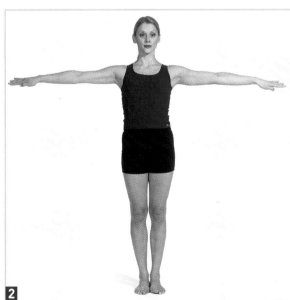
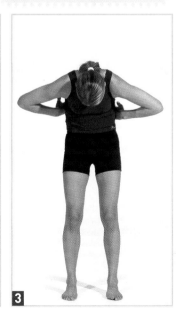

Criss-cross & loop

Target helps you to balance co-ordination between the right and left side of your body, and helps to get your body working within your Centreline. Improves concentration. It is important to focus on the same spot on a wall or in a mirror throughout the exercise.

Position stand upright, with your feet together or hip width apart. Look straight ahead.

Criss-cross steps

- focus on your Centreline.
- bring your right hand and left knee close to each other until they touch.
- focus on to your Centreline.
- change direction; bringing your left hand closer to your right knee.
- keep your eyes focused on one spot.
- repeat this 8 times to begin with.

Loop steps

- bring your left hand and left knee together.
- change over, bringing your right hand and right knee together.
- repeat this 8 times to begin with.

The most important part of this exercise is when the criss-cross movement changes to a loop. Make sure that at this moment you focus on your Centreline and that your eyes do not wander around. You will notice how the change becomes smoother as you practice – your balance and sense of Centreline will improve.

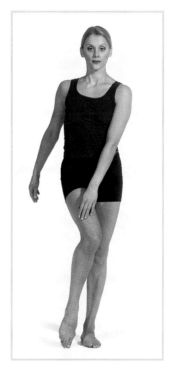

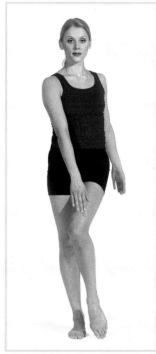

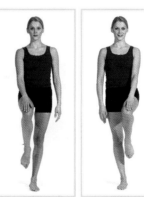

WARM-UP

half

Combine the Criss–Cross & Loop

- after you have completed the loop movement, change back to the criss-cross and start over again, repeating it 8 times.
- keep on changing between the two until you have completed each set of 8 movements 3 times.

Centreline Pull

WARM-UP

Target to balance your body towards its Centreline; to find a rhythm for your breathing.

Breathing Half Moon.

Position stand upright, with your feet together or hip width apart. Look straight ahead and hold your arms in front of your body. Bend your elbows, and put your hands together with your palms against each other.

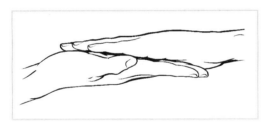

Steps

- ✴ inhale and bend your knees.

- ✴ exhale, straighten your legs and extend your right arm upwards, turning the palm of your hand up towards the ceiling; and turning the palm of your left hand towards the floor.

- ✴ inhale, bend your knees, and turn the palms of your hands to face each other; slowly bringing them closer until they are nearly touching.

- ✴ exhale, and this time extend your left arm upwards and right arm downwards.

- ✴ continue to repeat the sequence, alternating your hands.

- ✴ focus on keeping your eyes on the same spot in front of you.

- ✴ think about your Centreline.

tip
After repeating the movement several times you will find a good rhythm and flow. This movement also allows you to become aware of your Stabilising Points; the Navel Point and Diaphragm Point, and their movement in front of your spine.

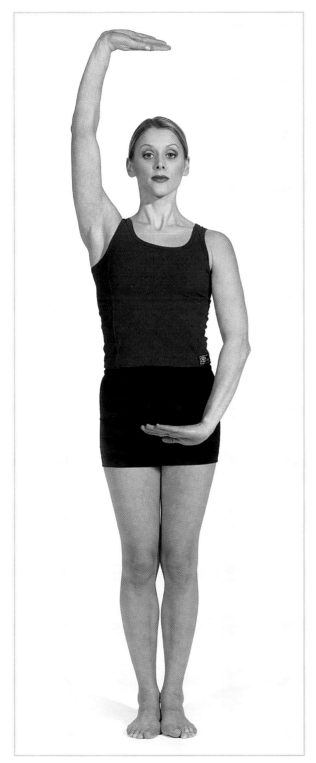

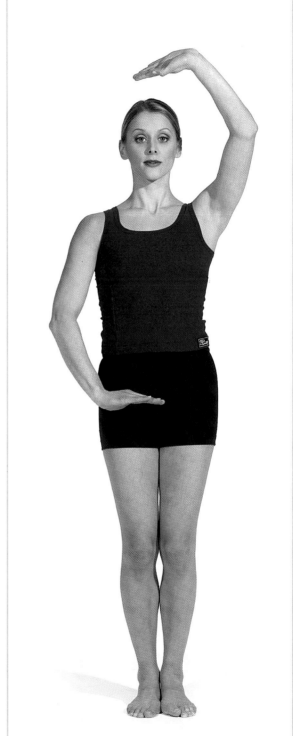

CENTERING EXERCISES

Dance of the eyes

You will already be familiar with this exercise from your first two days of preparatory work

Target to relax your eyes, and reach a deeper level of concentration; to find the 'centre' of your eyes.

Position sit upright and place your fingers on the focus point (the same position as described above) and close your eyes.

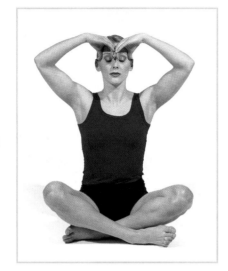
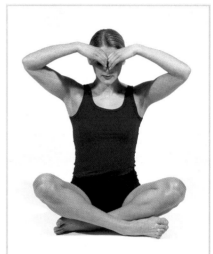

Steps

* move your eyes to the upper left corner; return to the centre
* move your eyes to the lower right corner; return to the centre
* move your eyes to the upper right corner; return to the centre
* move your eyes to the lower left corner; return to the centre

Travel through your Centreline

You will already be familiar with this exercise from your first two days of preparatory work

Target to focus on working from the 'inside out'. To find your Centreline, establish your Navel and Diaphragm Points, connect the floors of your body and learn to relax your body weight towards your spine.

Position lie on you back on the floor, with your knees bent. Place your heels hip width apart, and place your arms flat along the side of your body.

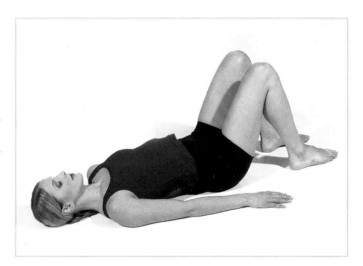

Steps

* visualise the space within your ribcage – it has a front, sides and a back. Drop your weight to the bottom of your ribcage. Feel how it falls onto the lowest part. In your mind move your area of focus, visualising your pelvis. Think about the shape of your pelvis from the inside out. The pelvis has sides, a back and is open at the front. It is built in two halves, which are connected to each other through the base of the spine.

* visualise the two sitting bones. Drop the weight on to the back of your pelvis – towards your sitting bones. In your mind move your area of focus to your spine. The spine begins almost from behind your eye level. From there it continues its way down through your neck to your ribcage, through your ribcage to your waist and pelvis, ending at the tailbone. Your spine has a front, which is at the moment facing towards the ceiling, and a back, which is

facing towards the floor. At the front, the vertebrae are rounded. Your Centreline travels in front of the spine – from the top of your head to your tailbone.

* relax your abdomen and feel the weight on the front of your spine.

* imagine there is a little man doing somersaults along the front of your spine. Each time a somersault is performed, you can sense the weight of your inner organs dropping onto that part of the spine.

* turn the tailbone towards your navel, and then away from your navel while visualising your Centreline.

Have a ball

You will already be familiar with this exercise from the 'consolidation' section of the book.

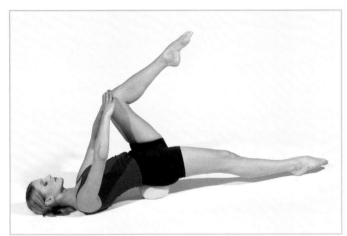

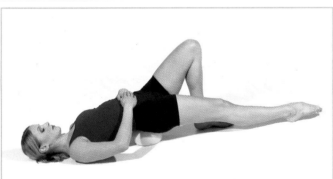

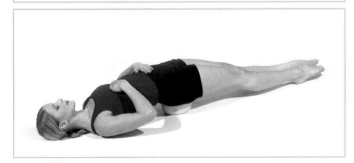

Preparation use a small soft ball as shown in the picture. If you don't have one of these it is just as good to use a tightly rolled towel or a small, tight cushion. It needs to be something that will both lift and support your pelvis while you are lying down.

Position lie on your back on the floor with your knees bent, and place your feet on the floor hip-width apart. Press your feet into the floor, and lift your pelvis up into the air. Place the ball underneath your tailbone. Tilt your tailbone, towards your Navel Point.

Breathing Half Moon

> **Note** Make sure the ball or towel is not underneath your lower back – it must be underneath your tailbone.

Steps (a)

* relax your eyes and focus on your Centreline.

* inhale using Half Moon breathing (see page 38).

* exhale and relax; move your Navel Point towards your spine, using your pelvic floor muscles to move your Navel Point closer to your Diaphragm Point.

* lift your left knee towards your chest (picture 1).

*Above all, listen to
your intuition and
common sense!*

- ✳ tilt your tailbone further towards your Navel Point.

- ✳ relax the Navel Point further towards your spine. Lower your left leg over the ball until your foot is on the floor. This is your Ground Point (picture 2).

- ✳ focus on relaxing your lower abdominals. Think about the space between the top of your leg and pelvis, and the idea that the bones are moving away from each other.

- ✳ if comfortable, straighten both your legs out (picture 3). Focus on slowing down your breathing, PAUSE at the end of exhalation.

- ✳ change legs, repeating the same movement.

tip
If you feel discomfort, make sure the ball is placed correctly, and that you are not tensing your back.

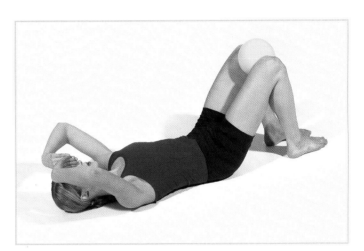

Note When your Diaphragm and Navel Point are relaxed towards your spine as you inhale, then your body weight is balanced towards your Centreline. If you feel that they are lifting upwards and away from your Centreline don't worry; the muscles around your waist and back are probably short. As your progress through the programme the weight of your Centre will move closer towards your spine.

Steps (b)

- ✳ bend both knees, and press your feet firmly on the floor, lift your pelvis off the ball and place the ball or towel between your knees.

- ✳ place your hands on the 'focus point of the eyes' (see page 25).

- ✳ roll through your spine; relax one vertebrae at a time onto the floor, following your Centreline – through your ribcage, waistline and pelvis until your pelvis reaches its neutral position; following the line of the floor (it is not tilted either forward or back). Squeeze the ball, and centre yourself.

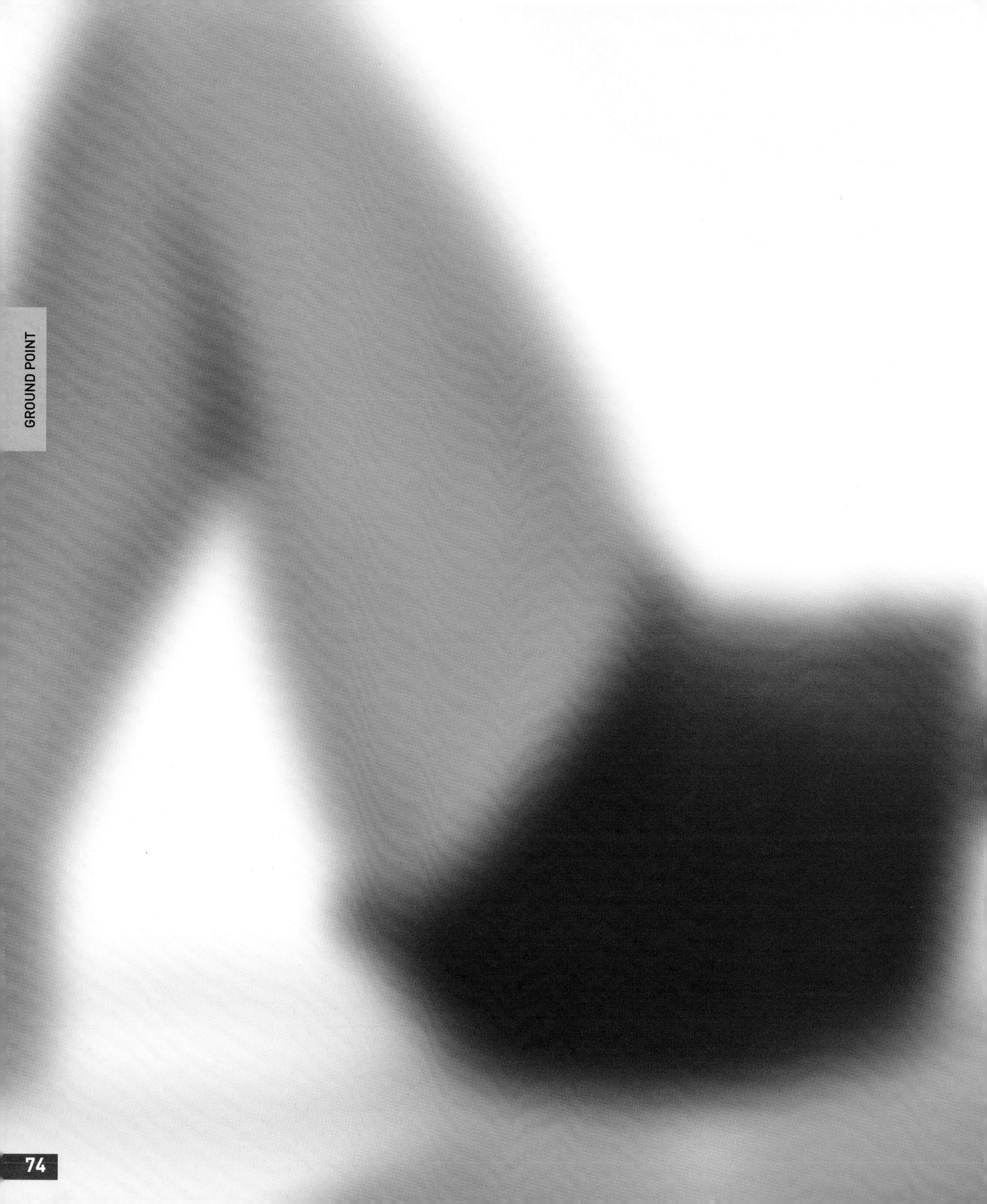

FIND YOUR
GROUND POINT

Find your Ground Point

You will already be familiar with this exercise from
your first two days of preparatory work

*First drop the weight,
and then transfer it*

Target to find your Ground Point.

Position lie on your back, keeping your back
straight. Bend your knees and place your
heels together, in line with your sitting bones.
Press your feet firmly into the ground,
observing how your lower back feels lighter.
    Release the pressure through your feet, and
feel the weight shift back to your lower back.

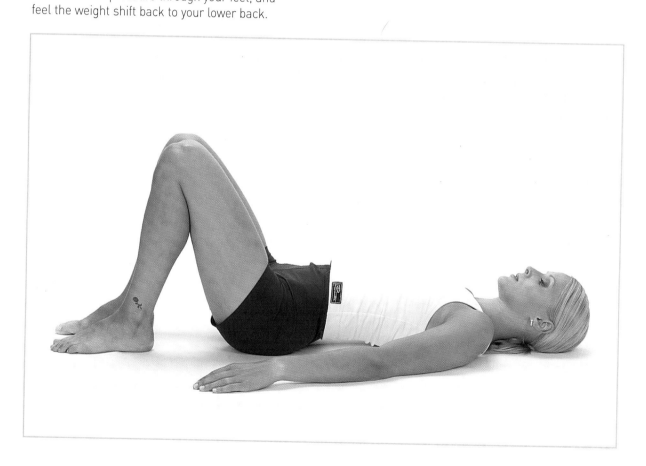

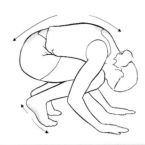

Rabbit stretch

You will already be familiar with this stretch from your first two days of preparatory work

Target to find your Ground Point; to master the use of gravity in your stretches.

Position crouch on the floor and arch your back forwards, bringing your knees towards your chest. Place your hands the floor and tilt your head down. Relax your body weight towards your heels.

Alternate between shifting your body weight backwards and forwards – first towards your hands and then back towards your feet. Explore the sense of the weight shifting from your feet to your hands and back to your feet again.

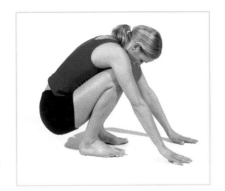

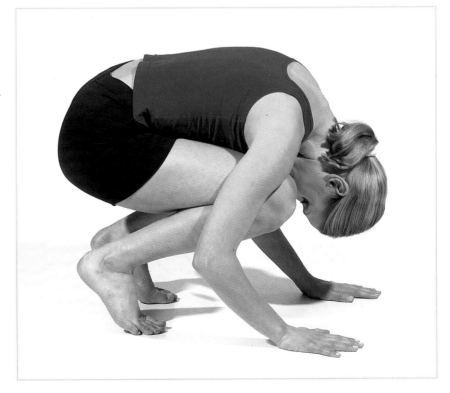

Toe stretch

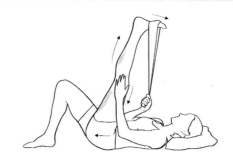

Target to focus on your Centreline; to realign your legs.

Breathing Half Moon.

Equipment band, scarf or belt.

Position lie on the floor and place a small cushion or rolled towel under your head. Place your feet on the floor and bend your knees. Release your neck by tilting your chin towards your chest. Lift your left leg towards the ceiling, using a band, scarf or towel. Start to straighten your raised left leg, but don't lock your knee. Grasp the scarf with your right hand as you do this. You can place your left hand on your forehead to create a focus point if you wish.

tip
Massage the web of your big toe with a firm touch for approximately 30 seconds – this will help to improve the overall balance of your body by aligning your foot with your pelvis.

Steps

* inhale and relax your eyes.

* exhale; and mentally travel through your Centreline – through your ribcage, waistline and pelvis to your tailbone.

* from here travel up, following the line of your outstretched leg at the back. When you reach your heel, push it towards the ceiling.

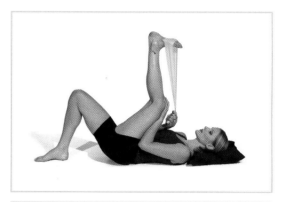

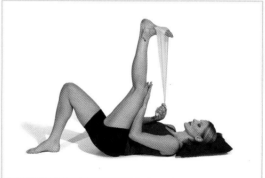

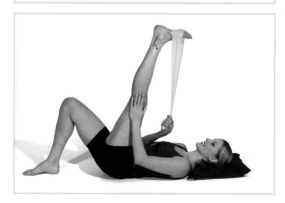

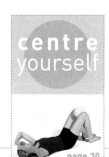

centre yourself page 30

GROUND POINT

* continue this visualisation, moving over the heel, across the arch of the foot and down the front of your leg from the toe. Aim to align your leg within your Centreline, keeping your heel and your knee in line with your hip. Keep the bottom of your foot flat towards the ceiling.

* exhale, PAUSE, and further open up the back of your knee, softly.

* repeat the visualisation and breathing.

* straighten the right leg on the floor next to the left leg, and feel the difference between the two.

* repeat the same movement with the right leg.

tip

Find your Ground Point by relaxing your body weight towards your sitting bones and your supporting leg on the floor.

After working on both legs, you will be able to find the Ground Point under your feet more easily, whether standing up or lying down.

Advanced Toe Stretch

Position if you find this movement fairly easy then you can move onto the advanced version. Instead of using a band or scarf, just grasp your big toe with your hand, and go through the same stages outlined above. Feel more; utilise the magic moment of the PAUSE (at the end of exhalation) in order to progress.

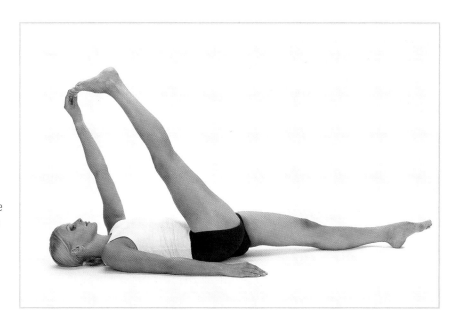

Triangle stretch

If you find this position difficult, start by working on the soft triangle stretch on page 82 first.

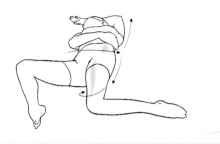

Muscle targets muscles around your waist, hip flexors and abdominals.

Breathing Half Moon.

Main effects increases the length of the waist; improves the shape of the waist; pulls the stomach in; relaxes the diaphragm; relieves tension in the lower back; reduces cellulite.

Targets when getting into this position, think about the round shape of the femoral bone at the top of your thigh, and how it is able to rotate inwards in your hip socket.

Position sit on the floor with your knees bent and your feet very wide apart. Lean back, supporting your body weight on your hands, with your fingers pointing forwards.

tip
Focus on your lower abdominal muscles.

Steps (a)

✳ roll your left leg towards your Centreline (rotate it inwards from the hip joint). Turn you right leg out.

✳ shift your body weight slightly towards the right hand side of your sitting bones, and allow the left side of your pelvis to lift off the floor (picture 1).

✳ bend your right arm and drop back onto your elbow, supporting your weight.

✳ drop your back onto the floor, allowing the right leg to relax – lift your right knee off the floor if you need to, ensuring that there is no pressure on the knee.

✳ finally, extend your left arm over your head, and turn your head to the right. Place your right hand over your left side of your ribcage (picture 2).

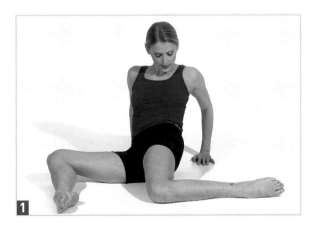

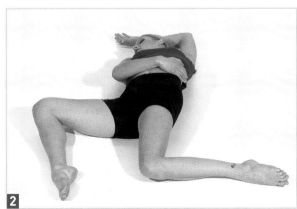

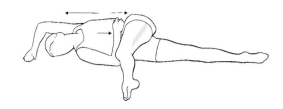

Steps (b)

* inhale, and focus on your Centreline; relax your abdominal muscles towards your spine.

* exhale, and create the stretch by moving your Diaphragm Point deeper towards your spine. PAUSE, and focus on your Navel Point; increasing the distance between your Navel Point and your tailbone. Move your left knee further towards the floor if you can, but don't force it.

* move your hands to your abdomen. As you inhale, resist the pressure of the breathing with your hands.

* exhale and pull the abdomen gently down towards your spine, and then up towards your ribs. Tilt your tailbone up towards your navel, keeping your buttocks relaxed. Feel the stretch in the very lowest part of your abdomen.

* PAUSE, and take your time before the next inhalation.

Steps (c)

* begin to move your left leg over the right leg until you are able to fully straighten it out.

* rotate your ribcage towards your left, extend your arm and turn your head towards the right.

* inhale towards the left side of your ribs

* roll onto your back, and repeat the whole sequence on the other side.

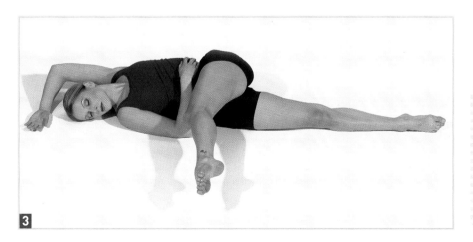

3

Note Use your torso as one unit to rotate the pelvis towards the left. If you feel that you need to ease the stretch a little, you can place a pillow under your lower back.

Soft triangle stretch

You may have to work on the length of the muscles at the front of your thighs and your hip flexors, until they are long enough for you to be able to reach the Traingle stretch on page 80.

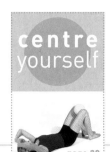

centre yourself

page 30

GROUND POINT

Position lie on your back with your knees bent, and place your feet on the floor with your legs wide apart. Lean back onto your arms.

Breathing Half Moon.

> **Note** Keep your weight focused towards your Navel Point, so that it feels heavy.

Steps

* inhale to prepare.
* exhale, and roll your left leg inwards, towards your Centreline; controlling the movement with your Abdominal Corset.
* PAUSE, and focus on your Navel Point, engaging your First Floor (see page 35).

* inhale, and return your left leg to its upright starting position.
* repeat the same movement on the other side.
* continue to alternate between the two legs; completing the movement approximately 3 times on each side.

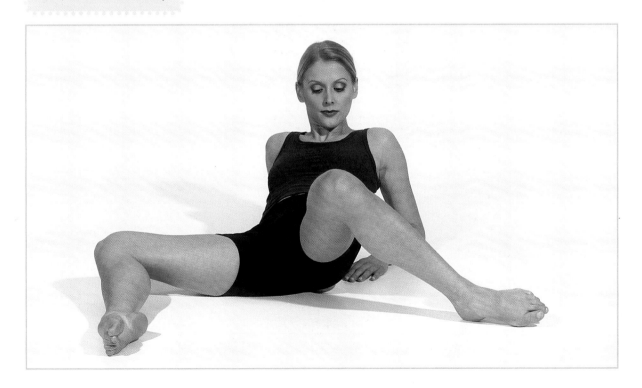

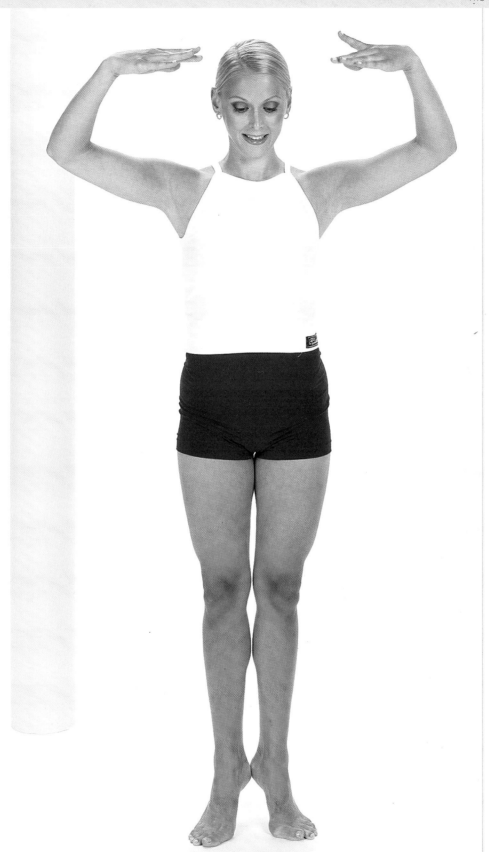

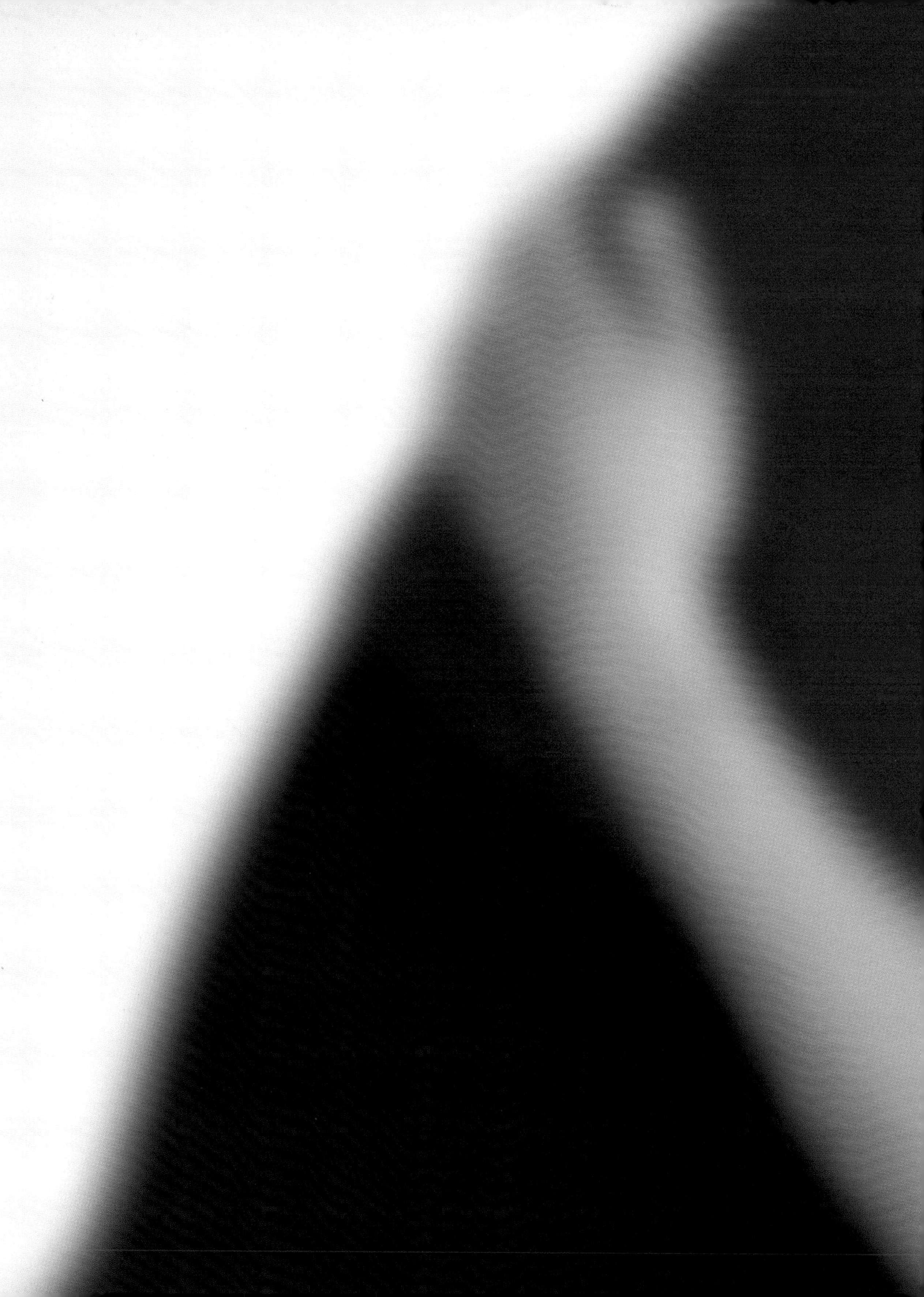

FIND YOUR
BREATHING PUMP

Bow stretch **on the floor**

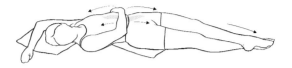

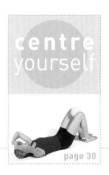
centre
yourself

page 30

Muscle targets muscles around waist, hip flexors and abdominals.

Breathing Half Moon.

Main effects to find your breathing pump; to lift your waist.

Position Lie on your back with your legs straight. Increase the distance between your ribcage and pelvis by tilting your left side of your ribcage away from your pelvis to create the shape of a 'bow'. Cross your left leg over your right leg, and extend your left arm over your head. Reach your right hand over your body to reach the lowest part of your ribcage on the left. Turn your head towards your right shoulder.

Steps

* focus on the left side of your lungs, and breathe into this area (just under your right hand). Focus on pulling your Diaphragm Point in towards your spine, and down towards your Navel Point.

* release the diaphragm when exhaling so it moves upwards. Stretch your left leg further away from your hip socket, and away from your Navel Point.

* PAUSE and allow your Abdominal Corset to sink deeper towards the centre of your body; allow your diaphragm to rise into its highest position.

* repeat the breathing sequence 3–5 times while holding this position – take your time!

* repeat the stretch on the other side.

tip
When inhaling, make sure you relax your neck and shoulders as much as possible – inhaling slowly will help you do this. Ensure that your breastbone expands outwards from your Centreline while you inhale.

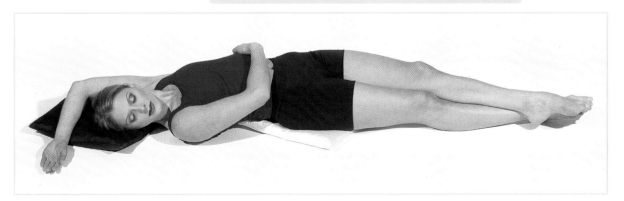

Bow stretch

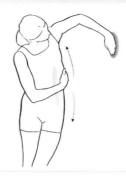

Muscle targets muscles around your waist, hip flexors and abdominals.

Main effects increase the length of the waist; to shape the waist; to pull the stomach in; to relax the diaphragm; to relieve tension in the lower back; to reduce cellulite.

Breathing Half Moon.

Position stand with your left side to a wall or door frame. Place the heel of your left foot on top of your right foot. Lift your left elbow upwards, rotating it from the shoulder. Place the palm of your hand flat against the wall with your fingers facing down at a height that feels comfortable. Create a 'bow' by lifting your ribcage up and away from your pelvis, and bending your supporting leg and arm a little. You have already assumed this position on the floor in the previous stretch. Turn your head towards your left shoulder. Place your right hand on the left side of your ribcage, at its lowest point.

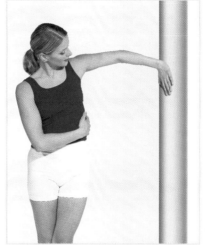

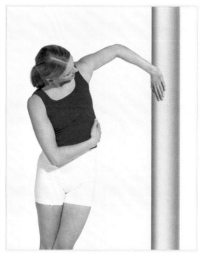

Steps

- focus on increasing the space between your pelvis and your ribcage.
- inhale to help you expand the side that you are stretching.
- exhale, and create the stretch as you PAUSE.
- allow your diaphragm to release, lifting your ribs away from your pelvis.

tip
If possible, look at your position in a mirror.

- increase the space between your ribs and your pelvis further by dropping your weight towards your Navel Point .
- continue with the Half Moon breathing a few times.
- repeat on other side.

Note keep your ribcage moving upwards and away from your pelvis; as you add more weight towards your Navel Point be careful not to concentrate the weight on your hand.

DEEP STRETCHES:
LEGS, PELVIS & BUTTOCKS

Humming bird stretch

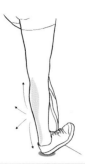

Muscle targets calf muscles, Achilles tendon.

Main effects to improve circulation to the legs; to shape the lower part of the legs and knees; to slim the ankle.

Breathing Half Moon.

Position stand sideways within a doorframe; flex your right foot upwards placing your toes against the frame with the weight on your heel. Keep your leg straight, but do not lock your knee. Place your left foot half a stride behind your right, and relax your toes. Place your hands either side of the doorframe. Keep your torso upright and forward.

Steps

✳ inhale.

✳ exhale, and start to lift the heel of your left foot off the floor.

✳ maintain your upright position, and create the stretch by shifting your whole body (as one unit) towards the wall, transferring your body weight into the right calf, and placing your left foot on top of the right.

✳ use your arms on the doorframe to pull your body forward. Keep the right leg passive. PAUSE before your next inhalation.

✳ try to wiggle the toes of your right foot to help you feel the muscle connections between your toes and your calves.

✳ repeat on other side.

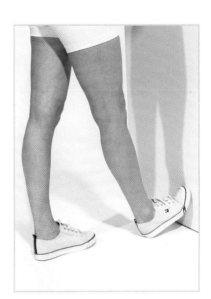

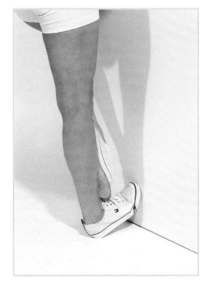

tip

To stretch a deeper layer of the calf muscles and the Achilles tendon, start with both your knees bent. Create the stretch by extending the right leg first, pushing against your Ground Point. Once you feel the stretch increasing, lift your left leg off the floor, and place it over the top of your right foot.

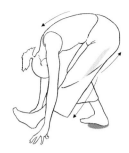

Swan dive

Muscle targets hamstrings.

Main effects to lift the buttocks; to change the tilt of your pelvis and your back; to release lower back tension; to connect with the leg muscles.

Breathing Half Moon.

Position stand facing a wall, placing the toes of your left foot against the wall, with your heel on the floor. Place the right leg one good stride behind the left and tilt your torso forward. Place your hands on the floor, pushing the floor away to create a Ground Point to support your body weight. Keep both legs bent, drop your head down and relax your neck.

Note In this position you will feel a strong sensation of the nerves. Use your Ground Point to push against the floor, and ease this feeling.

tip
This is a difficult position, especially for beginners. Using blocks or a support of some kind under each hand will enable you to balance without straining to reach the floor.

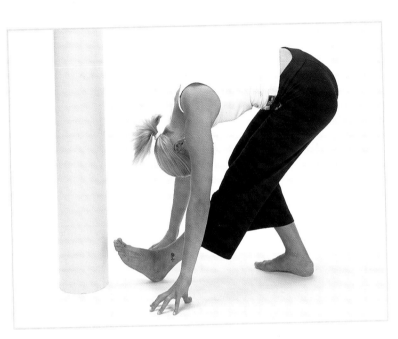

Steps

* focus on the muscles at the back of your leg; your hamstrings and your calf muscles.

* inhale.

* as you exhale, create the stretch by straightening your left leg and gently pointing your toes upwards, applying more body weight to the muscles at the back of the thigh.

* deepen or ease the stretch by bending or straightening the supporting leg. As you begin to straighten it, push your heel into the floor to further lengthen your hamstring.

* move your right leg further back, and repeat the above.

* as the calf muscles and hamstrings at back of the knee begin to lengthen, you may further straighten your left leg, shifting more of your body weight forward.

* repeat on the other side.

Lizard stretch

Muscle targets front of thigh; hip flexor.

Main effects to change the shape of the front of your legs; to adjust the tilt of your pelvis.

Equipment a support, such as a chair, low table or wall.

Position kneel on the floor and bend your right leg in front of your body, creating a 90-degree angle, keep your foot flat on the floor. Extend your left leg out behind you, rotating it slightly inwards from your hip joint. Place your hands on the support, transferring some of your weight through your hands (Ground Point) to ease up the pressure in the pelvic area. Engage your First Floor (pelvic floor) (see page 35).

Note Due to the depth of these muscles, it is important during exhalation to engage the pelvic floor. You can recognise it engaging when you feel a lift in your lower abdominal area.

Steps

* focus on the deep muscles of the hip and front thigh areas.

* shift your bodyweight around the thigh; outside, middle, inside and so on. Settle into the position you feel is working best for you. (Remember as your stretches increase, the focus for the stretch will naturally travel to different areas.)

* inhale.

* keep your hand on the support, exhale, and create the stretch at the end of the exhalation. PAUSE. Apply more body weight gradually through your pelvis to increase the stretch.

* continue the stretch with the flow of your breathing.

* repeat on other side.

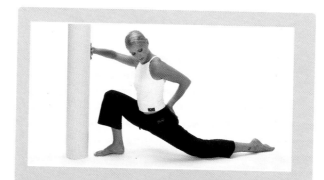

tip
To increase your focus you can place your left hand on your left buttock, slightly above your tailbone.

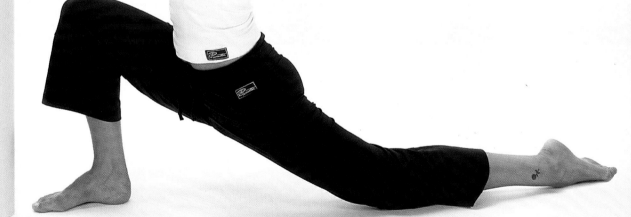

half

Swan stretch

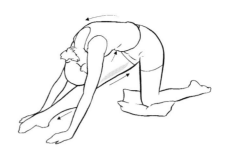

LEGS, PELVIS & BUTTOCKS

half

Muscle targets hamstrings.

Main effects to lift the buttocks; to change the tilt of your pelvis and your back; to release lower back tension.

Position you can continue into this position from the Lizard Stretch (page 92) by bringing your left leg forward, and extending your right leg out in front of you. Keep your right leg as straight as possible, but don't lock your knee. Keep it bent at the knee if it is easier. Bend your torso forward over your Diaphragm Point.

Steps

* focus on your hamstrings.

* inhale.

* exhale, PAUSE and create the stretch by slowly straightening your right leg; work towards your Ground Point by transferring the weight of your torso forward.

* once you are able to feel the stretch, deepen it by repeating the above; gradually applying more body weight through the back of your thigh muscles.

* repeat on the other side.

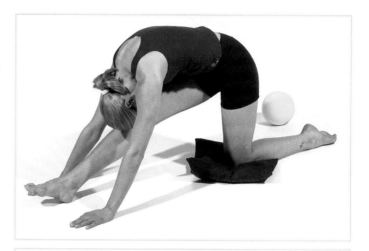

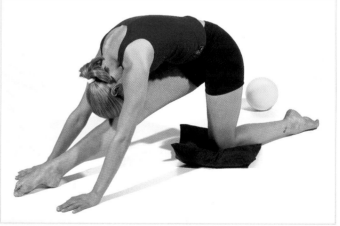

tip

This is a difficult position, especially for beginners. Using blocks or a support of some kind under each hand will enable you to balance without straining to reach the floor.

Note Push your heel into the floor to achieve a controlled straightening of your leg. Continue to tilt your tailbone away from your navel. As your hamstring lengthens, you may gradually decrease the bend in your right knee.

Swan rotation

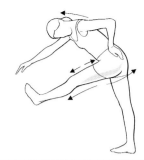

Muscle targets outer thigh.

Main effects to alter the shape of the legs, particularly their straightness.

Breathing Half Moon.

Position stand next to a chair or table and extend your left leg diagonally in front of you. Rotate your right supporting leg inwards. Lean your torso and right arm forward diagonally, towards your left leg. Tilt your tailbone away from your navel.

Steps

* focus on the outside of your thigh.

* inhale.

* exhale, PAUSE, and create the stretch. Slowly turn your torso to the left, leaning slightly forward. Make sure you give yourself enough time to feel the stretch on your outer thigh.

* repeat on the other side.

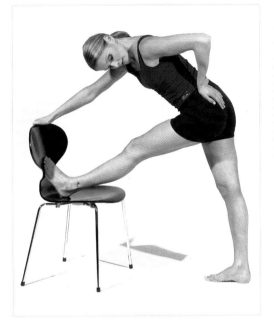

Note For many people this outside leg muscle is a blind spot. Use visualisation to connect with the muscle, and use your Ground Points to increase the weight through the muscle. Be prepared to spend time getting this stretch right.

VARIATION

You can do this stretch while kneeling, placing your arm on a support. If you are not able connect with this stretch, first focus on lengthening your hamstrings and the muscles at the front of your thigh. Use the Swan Stretch to work on your hamstrings, and the Lizard Stretch to work on the front of your thigh.

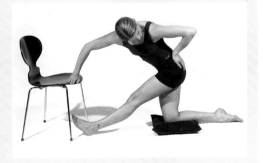

Sitting stork stretch

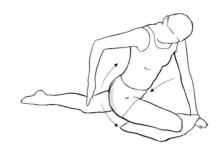

Muscle targets buttocks.

Main effects to improve the position of your pelvis; to release tension in the lower back; to lift the buttock line; to increase circulation; to help reduce cellulite.

Breathing Half Moon.

Position kneel on the floor in a lunge position, with your right leg bent in front of you, and your left leg extended behind. Place your hands either side of your body for support. Turn the knee of your right leg out to the right on the floor, moving your foot across your Centreline (pictures 1 and 2); sit on your left buttock. Keep your left leg extended behind you, and rotate it slightly inwards from the hip. Lean your torso slightly forward, bending your arms (picture 3).

Steps

☀ focus on the deep buttock muscles and the sitting bone area on the left side.

☀ use breathing to open up your lower back.

☀ create the stretch while exhaling. Bend your arms and lower your torso to apply additional weight through the part of the buttock you are working on.

☀ repeat on other side.

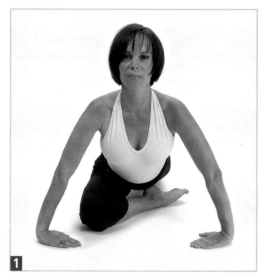

1

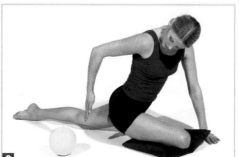

2

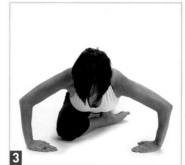

3

Standing stork stretch

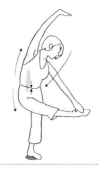

centre yourself

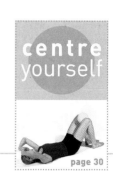

page 30

Muscle targets buttocks, hip flexors.

Main effects to change the tilt of the pelvis; to open the lower back; to lift the buttock line; to increase circulation; to help reduce cellulite.

Breathing Half Moon.

Position stand in front of a supporting surface like a chair or table, lifting your right leg up in front of you at waist height or slightly lower, bending your knee. Rest your foot on the support, and drop the knee to the right, rotating your leg from the hip socket until the knee faces outwards, but keep your pelvis facing forward. Place your hands on the support, and curve the upper body over your leg, controlling your weight with your hands, and assuming the 'bow' shape.

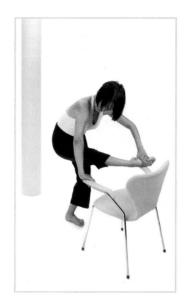

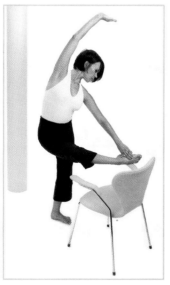

Steps

✳ focus on the muscles around your waistline, and the buttock muscles (your sitting bone area) of the right raised leg.

✳ inhale and allow your lower back to expand.

✳ exhale, and focus on your Abdominal Corset, curving your upper back further into a bow shape.

✳ PAUSE, and feel the stretch by creating a opposite movement, dropping your right knee further down. You will feel the stretch in your buttocks.

✳ deepen the stretch by rotating your torso towards the right, focusing more of your body weight through the left supporting leg.

✳ repeat on the other side.

Note Take your time with this stretch. The muscles you are working on are deep and strong, so it may take 10–20 seconds before you can even feel them. Take more of your weight through the foot of the standing leg.

This a very good stretch for mobilising your waistline and opening up your lower back. Lift your ribcage away from your hip, so it moves up and over your Diaphragm Point. Focus on your waistline.

Box split stretch

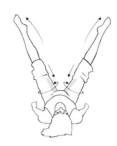

Muscle targets inner thighs.

Main effects to improve the position of your pelvis; to lift the buttocks.

Breathing Half Moon.

Position lie on your back, with your legs and bottom up against a wall. Make sure you keep your back flat on the floor. Open your legs into a V-shape position, rotating them out from the hip sockets. Relax your weight on to the back of your pelvis.

Steps

* focus on the inner thigh muscles.

* inhale.

* exhale, and connect your First Floor (pelvic floor) with your Navel and Diaphragm Points. Relax your tailbone towards the floor (increasing the distance from your Navel Point). Widen the V-shape.

* follow the rhythm of your breathing and work towards taking a substantial amount of time with this stretch (5-8 minutes). Remember to relax!

tip

If you feel uncomfortable, bring the inner thighs closer to each other and then release back down. Repeat this when you feel you need to.

You can also apply additional weight by placing your hands on your inner thighs and alternate between gently pressing your legs down, and then up against your hands.

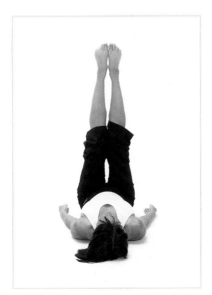

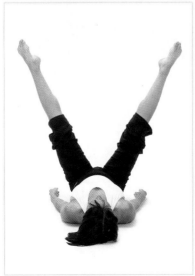

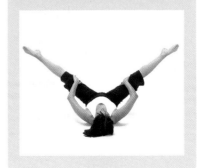

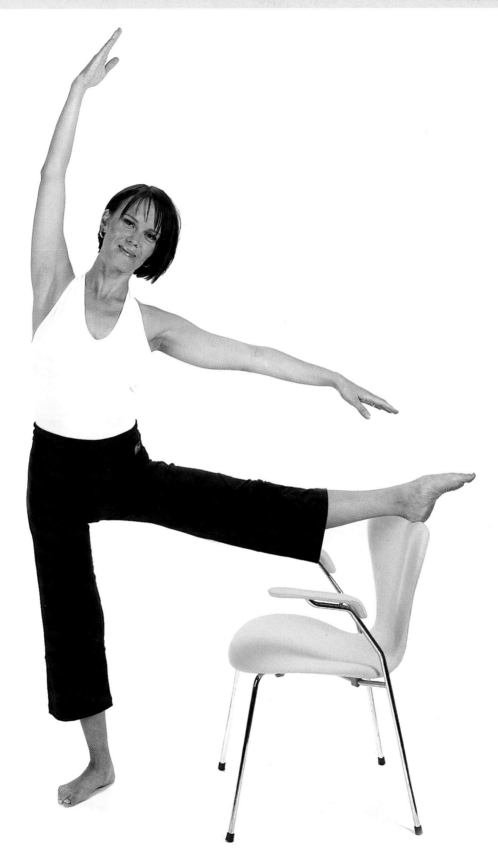

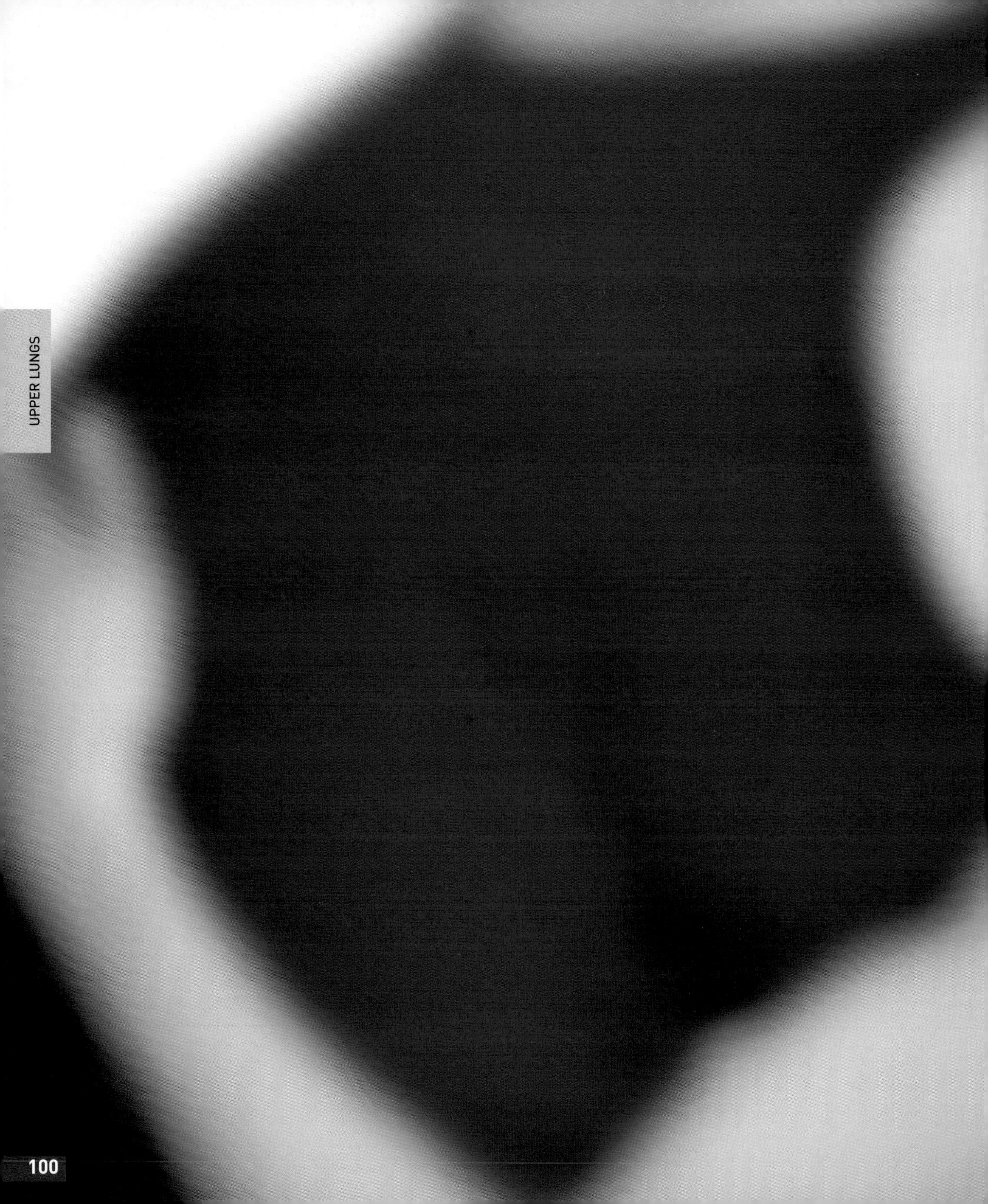

FIND YOUR
UPPER LUNGS

Rising Sun breathing

Target to find your upper lungs.

Equipment small soft ball, pillow or rolled towel.

Breathing Half Moon.

Position sit on the floor, placing a small ball or rolled towel below your shoulder blades. Lean forwards on the ball, bending your knees and interlocking your fingers behind your head. Initiate the move from you abdominals – do not use your hands to pull your head forwards.

Steps

* inhale towards the lower part of your ribcage.

* exhale, and connect the Floors of your body. Hold the weight towards your Centreline, and slowly lean back over the ball as if you were unwinding your spine, until the top of your head reaches a cushion or the floor.

* inhale using Rising Sun breathing, and open your elbows. Focus on filling your upper lungs and allowing your ribcage to expand.

* exhale, PAUSE, and close your elbows together.

* stay in this position for as long as you feel comfortable; inhaling and exhaling.

* using your Abdominal Corset, lift your head, shoulders and upper back over the ball into the starting position.

* inhale towards your middle back.

* stay in this position inhaling and exhaling for as long as it feels comfortable. Otherwise, repeat the up and down movement 3 times.

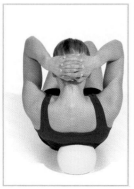 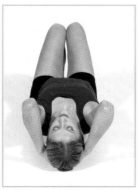 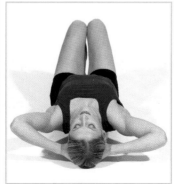 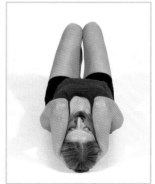

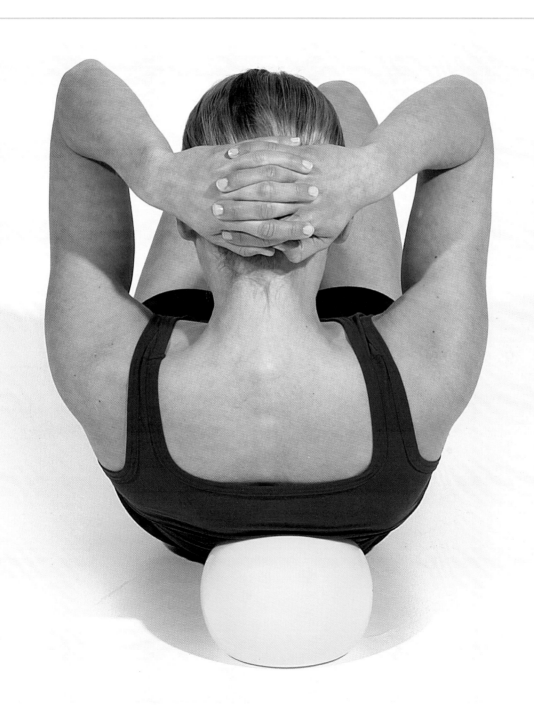

DEEP STRETCHES: CHEST

Butterfly stretch

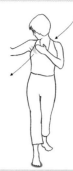

Muscle targets chest.

Main effects to open the chest and the shoulder line; to lift the breasts and tone the underarms; to expand your breathing capacity; to increase circulation to the head; to reduce tiredness, neck and shoulder tension and headaches.

Breathing Rising Sun.

Position using a doorframe or pillar, place your right forearm flat against it, with your elbow bent and your fingers pointing up. Step forward with your right foot, shifting your weight onto it. Bend your knees slightly. Place your left hand onto your chest to help you focus on the stretch.

Steps

✳ focus on the chest and the shoulder area.

✳ inhale using Rising Sun breathing.

✳ exhale, PAUSE, and lean further forward, taking the muscle to its new length by bending your legs a little more.

✳ deepen the stretch by rotating your torso and head away from your right arm, keeping the control between your Navel point and your Diaphragm Point. Follow the flow of your breathing.

✳ repeat on the other side.

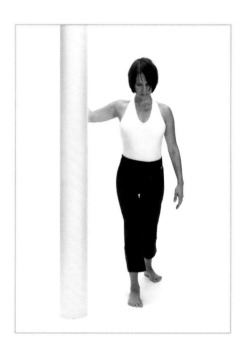

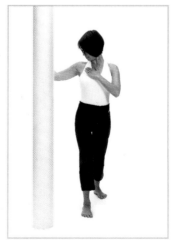

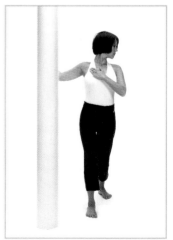

Kneeling butterfly stretch

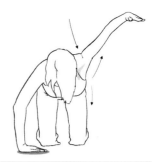

Muscle targets chest.

Main effects to open the chest and shoulders; to lift the breasts and tone the underarms; to expand the breathing capacity; to increase circulation to the head; to reduce tiredness, neck and shoulder tension and headaches.

Position kneel next to a chair or a table (slightly higher than torso level). Keeping your knees in line with your hips, lift your left arm onto the chair or table, so it is placed slightly forwards and higher than your chest.

Steps

* focus on your chest.
* inhale using Rising Sun breathing.
* exhale, PAUSE, and create the stretch by leaning your torso forward. By bending your supporting arm (Ground Point), you can gradually apply more body weight through the chest.

* stay with the stretch and deepen it by focusing on exhaling for longer, holding the PAUSE before you inhale again.
* repeat on the other side.

Note As you deepen this stretch, allow your shoulder blades to move down along your back to help open up your chest and relax your head. Focus on the deeper layer of chest muscles.

Experiment with slightly altering the position of your arm in order to feel the stretch at a different point.

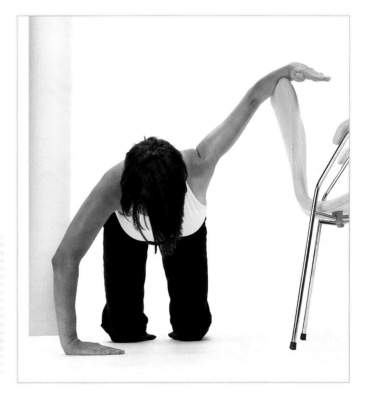

Swallow bird I

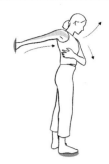

Muscle targets biceps.

Main effects to shape the arms; to broaden the shoulder line; to relax the shoulders; to improve circulation to the neck, shoulders, arms and hands.

Breathing Rising Sun.

Position stand beside a wall or pillar. Rotate your right arm backwards from the shoulder, placing your palm against the wall at around shoulder height. Lean towards the thumb side of your palm. Step forward onto your left leg, shifting the weight onto it. Bend your knees slightly if it is comfortable to do so. Be aware of your Centreline. Allow your head to relax.

Steps

✴ focus on your biceps, located at the front of your arm.

✴ inhale using Rising Sun breathing.

✴ exhale, PAUSE, and create the stretch by rotating your torso away from your arm. Readjust into your Centreline if necessary.

✴ turn your feet gently away from your arm.

✴ deepen the stretch by relaxing into a breathing rhythm, and further rotating your torso and legs away from your arm.

✴ repeat on the other side.

Note 1. Stay close enough to the wall to be able to increase or decrease the weight applied through your arm. Keep your shoulders back throughout the stretch.

Note 2. The bicep is a complex muscle in terms of ligament connections, so you must use visualisation to connect. Once you can clearly feel the muscle, work slowly to deepen your stretch.

After you have rotated your body as far as possible, you can also take the stretch further by bending your knees while keeping your arm straight. Make sure you don't lock your elbow as you work your way through the muscle.

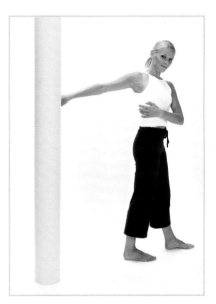

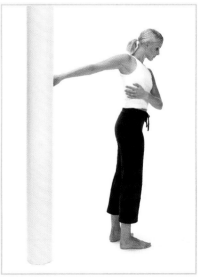

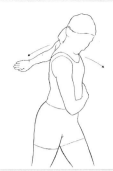

Swallow bird II

Muscle targets biceps.

Main effects to shape the arms; to broaden the shoulder line; to relax the shoulders; to improve circulation to the neck, shoulders, arms and hands.

Breathing Rising Sun.

Position: assume a similar position as in Swallow Bird I, but rotate your arm so that the back of your hand is against the wall. Step forward with the leg of the *same* side. Work through in the same way as the previous stretch.

Steps

* focus on your biceps, located at the front of your arm.

* inhale using Rising Sun breathing.

* exhale, PAUSE, and create the stretch by rotating your torso away from your arm. Readjust into your Centreline if necessary.

* turn your feet gently away from your arm.

* deepen the stretch by relaxing into a breathing rhythm, and further rotating your torso and legs away from your arm.

* repeat on the other side.

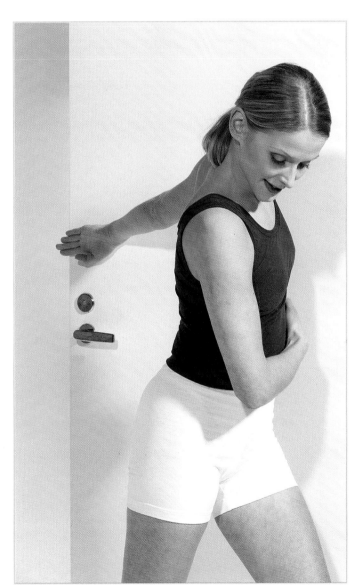

CHEST

109

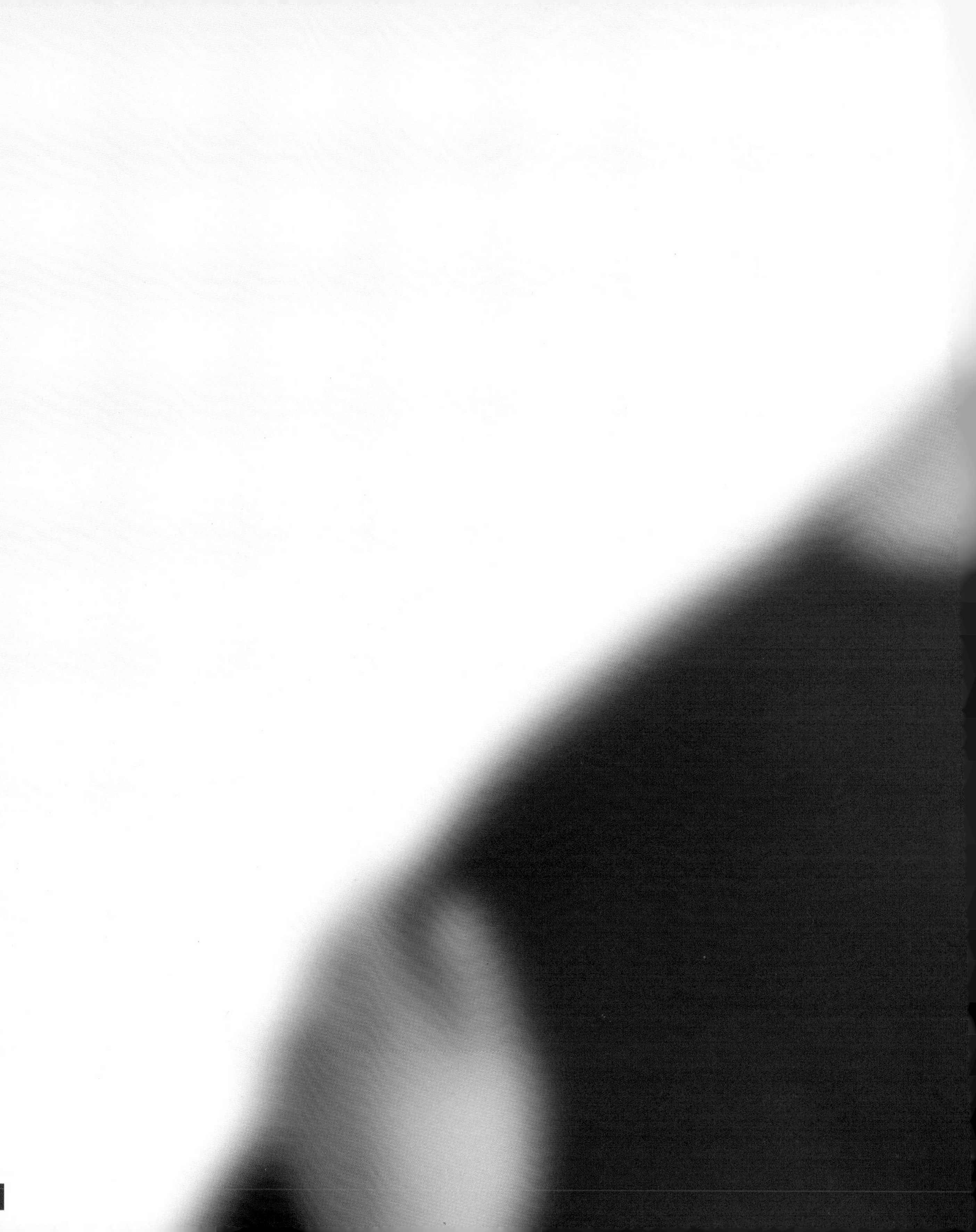

DEEP STRETCHES: BACK AND NECK

Somersault stretch

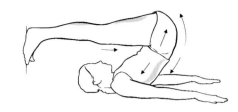

Muscle targets back and neck.

Main effects to lift your back; to shape your waistline; to pull your stomach in; to lift your chest; to reduce tension in the back; to alleviate tiredness.

Breathing Half Moon.

Position lie on your back with your head at arm's length from a wall or support. Pull your shoulders down and extend your arms forwards, pushing gently onto the floor. Bring your knees to your chest and move them apart. Breathe out and roll your legs over your head – initiating this movement from your tailbone. Place your feet on the wall and relax your chest towards the back of your ribs.

Steps

✳ inhale and focus on your upper back.

✳ exhale, PAUSE, and engage your abdominal corset. Relax the weight of your chest towards your shoulder blades.

✳ create the stretch by gently pushing your feet against the wall, and your hands into the floor (your Ground Points).

✳ lift your pelvis away from your ribcage, increasing the distance between your Navel Point and your Diaphragm Point.

✳ deepen the stretch by curving the tailbone towards your Navel point. This will increase the space between each vertebrae and release the muscles between your shoulder blades.

✳ stay in the stretch long enough to feel the stretch travelling down towards the lower back area and different parts of your back.

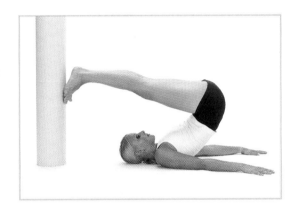

Note To benefit from this stretch, you need to have enough mobility in your lower back. If you find this position difficult, then don't force it. Instead, move onto the next stretch. As you progress through the programme, you may find that you are able to get into this position more easily.

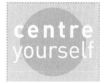
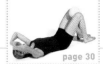
centre
yourself
page 30

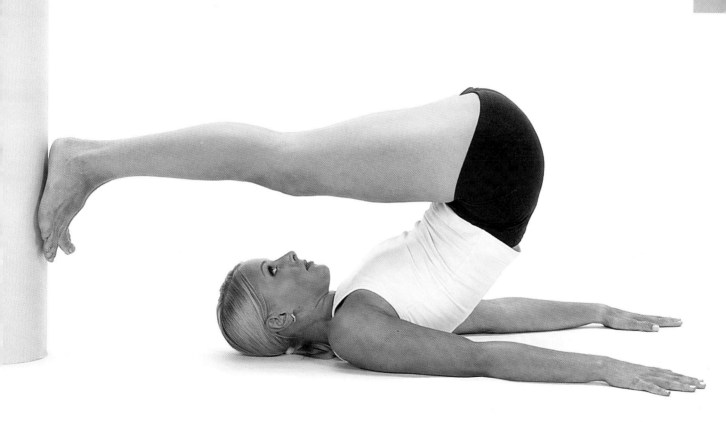

Snake charmer

Muscle targets muscles between your shoulder blades.

Main effects to increase circulation to the neck and face; to lift the face and neck; to release tension in the neck, shoulder and upper back area; to improve posture.

Breathing Rising Sun.

Position sit cross-legged on the floor or on a chair, keeping your back straight. Extend both arms down, with palms facing up, and cross the right over the left. Lift your right arm with your left, keeping the elbows crossed. Place your left hand on your right wrist, palms facing each other. Tilt your head to the left, and keep your right arm totally relaxed and passive. Relax your shoulders.

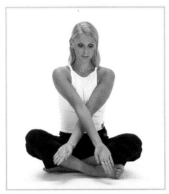

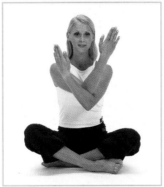

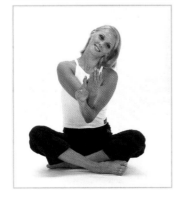

Steps

* focus on the muscles between your shoulder blades.

* inhale, focusing your breathing on your upper back.

* exhale, PAUSE, and create the stretch by actively using your left hand to press your right arm down towards the floor. Relax your upper chest and drop your shoulders further down.

* continue deepening the stretch by keeping your right arm passive as you slowly lift it up and down with the left arm. Gently press your right arm further down with your left hand as you pause at the end of exhalation.

* repeat using the opposite arm.

Note The upright positioning of your back is important. If you are sitting on a chair or against a wall, using a pillow against your lower back may help. If you find it difficult to maintain a straight back position, do the stretch standing against a wall with your feet in line with your hips.

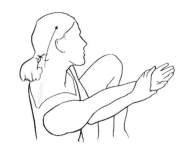

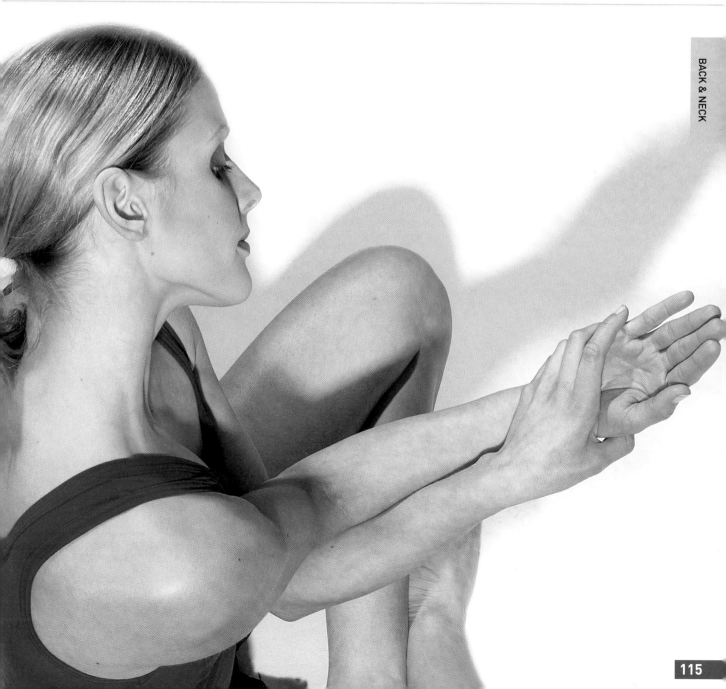

Tall crane stretch I

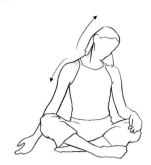

Muscle targets muscles at the side of your neck.

Main effects to increase circulation to the neck and face; to lift the face and neck; to release tension in the neck, shoulder and upper back area; to improve posture.

Breathing Rising Sun

Position sit upright in a cross-legged position, or on a chair. Relax your shoulders back and lift your chest upwards. Extend your right arm to the side, placing your hand on the floor with your palm facing up. Tilt your head to the left, lifting your cheek towards the ceiling. Relax your left arm.

Note Leading with your head, curve your torso to the left to further deepen the stretch. Ensure you keep your shoulders relaxed back.

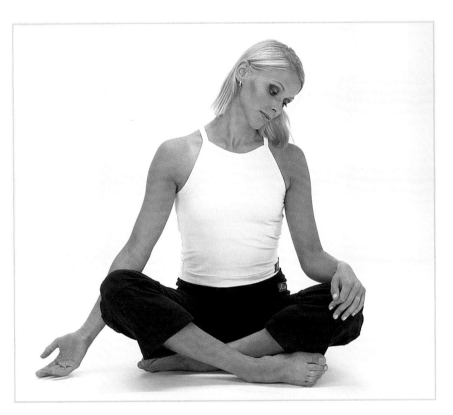

Steps

* focus on the right side of the neck.

* inhale.

* create the stretch by pushing your right arm out and slightly behind you. Further relax your head to the left.

* exhale, emptying the upper part of your lungs. PAUSE, keep your head in this relaxed position and deepen the stretch by slowly extending and lowering your right arm in slight movements.

* repeat on the other side.

Tall crane stretch II

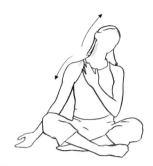

Muscle targets the back and side neck muscles.

Main effects to increases circulation to the neck and face; to lift the face and neck; to release tension in the neck, shoulder and upper back area; to improve posture.

Breathing Rising Sun.

Position sit cross-legged on the floor with a straight back. Assume the same position as before, extending your right arm to the side, placing your hand on the floor with your palm facing up, and tilting your head to the left, lifting your cheek towards the ceiling.

This time, place your left hand on your right collarbone.

Note Using your left hand to gently pull on the collarbone area helps to emphasize opening the right side of your neck.

Steps

* focus on the neck muscles running along the right side of your jaw line down to your collarbone.

* inhale.

* create the stretch by relaxing your head to the left and using your hand to gently pull down on the collarbone area. Feel the opening of the side of your neck.

* exhale, PAUSE, and deepen the stretch further by lifting your right cheek further towards the ceiling.

* repeat on the other side.

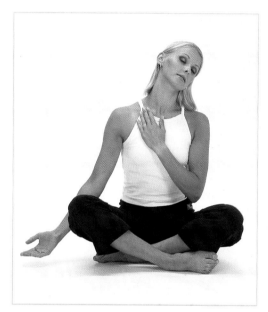

tip
If you would like to progress with this stretch, gently push your right arm further towards the floor, slightly behind your body. Experiment with using both hands on the muscles of the collarbone area to deepen the stretch.

Swan neck stretch

Muscle targets back of the neck; shoulders and upper back.

Main effects to increase circulation to the neck and face; to lift the face and neck; to release tension in the neck, shoulder and upper back area; to improve posture.

Breathing Rising Sun.

Position sit cross-legged and upright. Tilt your head slightly down (chin down to your chest). Interlock your fingers and place both hands behind your head. Bring your elbows together. Allow your neck, arms and upper back to be passive.

Steps

* focus on the back of your neck.

* inhale, focusing on breathing between the shoulder blades.

* create the stretch as you exhale, using the weight of your arms to bring your chin closer to your chest, increasing the curve of your upper back.

* fully empty the upper part of your lungs, engaging your abdominal corset to help you do this. Allow the pressure of the next inhalation to further deepen your stretch.

* work towards spending a good length of time on this stretch (at least 3 minutes).

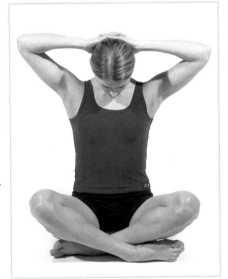

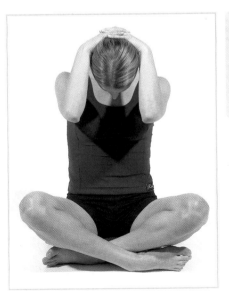

Note If this stretch feels as though it is creating too much pressure, ease it up whenever you feel you need to as you work towards a deeper stretch.
   Try varying the position of your head slightly to the right and left.

tip
Don't force your head down using your hands. Gently allow the weight of your arms to increase.

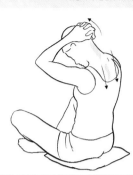

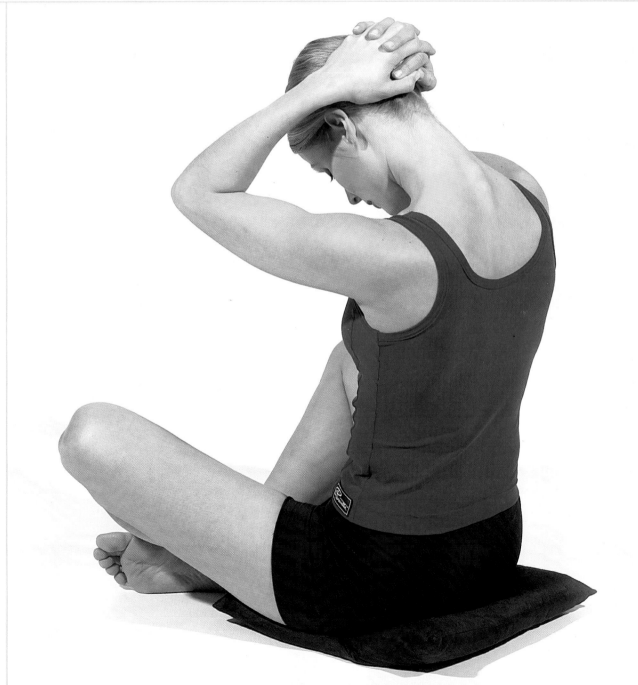

Otter stretch

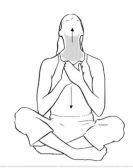

Muscle targets upper back and neck.

Main effects to increase circulation to the neck and face; to lift the face and neck; to release tension in the neck, shoulder and upper back area; to improve posture.

Breathing Rising Sun.

Position sit cross-legged and upright. Roll your shoulders back and relax them. Lift your chest up. Lengthen the front of your neck by slightly lifting your chin upward but do not close off the back of the neck. Place both your hands at the centre of your collarbone area, one on top of the other.

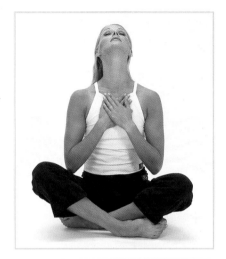

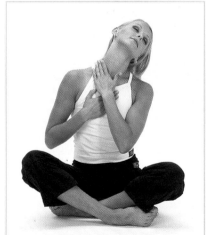

Steps

* focus on the neck muscles running from the top of your chest to your lower jaw line.

* inhale, and use your hands on your collarbone area to pull your neck muscles down. Feel them sliding over your collarbone, and further lift your chin upwards.

* exhale, PAUSE, further deepening the stretch. Feel the stretch at the top of your throat by swallowing.

* continue focusing on the side of your jaw by turning your head slightly to alternate sides.

Note By swallowing, you may become aware of the amount of tension you carry in the throat area underneath your chin. This stretch is suitable for addressing the tightness of the upper throat that can result in a double chin.

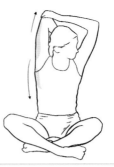

Sitting bat stretch

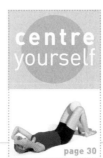

centre yourself

page 30

Muscle targets triceps.

Main effects to shape your arms; to relax the shoulders; to broaden the shoulder line; to open up the back.

Breathing Rising Sun.

Position sit cross-legged and upright. Raise your right arm and rotate in from the elbow, initiating the movement from your shoulder blade. Drop your hand to between your shoulder blades, keeping your elbow back. Allow your shoulder blade to drop down. Keeping your waist lifted, turn your head slightly to the left and focus your body weight through your right tricep.

tip
Keeping your shoulder blades down and relaxing your chest will help to isolate the triceps during this stretch.

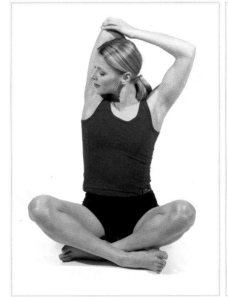

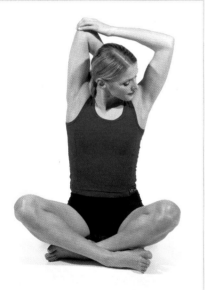

Steps

* focus on the triceps.

* inhale.

* exhale, PAUSE, creating the stretch by gently pushing your right elbow down towards your shoulder blade using your left hand, keeping your right arm passive.

* deepen the stretch by rotating your head and torso towards the left.

* hold the stretch, following the rhythm of your breathing.

* repeat using the other arm.

Note As the stretch deepens, imagine the shoulder blade gradually moving down the back and separating from the arm, lengthening the triceps as it does.

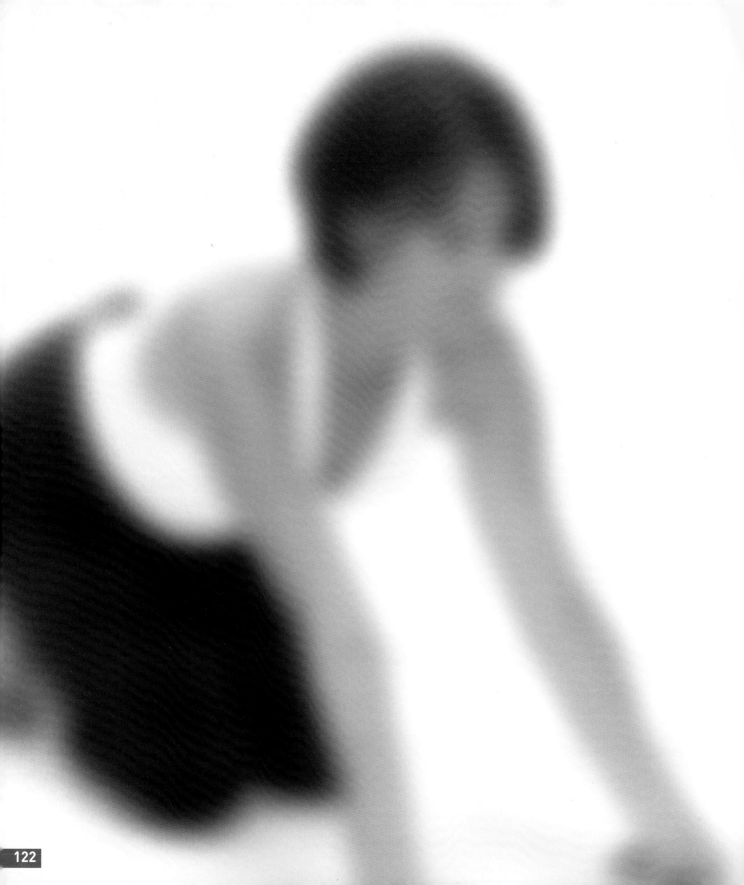

STRETCH AND STABILISING BANKS

STRETCH BANK

Congratulations! – you have now reached the end of the official programme. This part gives you some stretches that you may like to use to alternate your programme at a later stage. They may not be relevant to you during the 4 week programme, as you will be busy familiarising yourself with your body and working towards a deeper stretch. However, as you start to think about ways to incorporate stretches into your everyday life, you may wish to explore these positions, and work on them in the future if they help you achieve you long-term aims. Use them in your own time!

FLAMINGO STRETCH

GIBBON STRETCH

WINDSURFER STRETCH

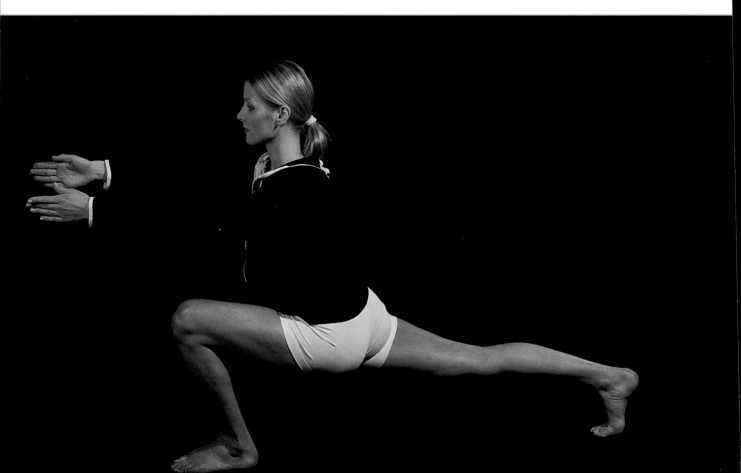

STABILISING BANK

Whenever you stand in an upright position or move, there are three main areas of your body that you need to stabilise to free yourself from tension:

* pelvis
* waist
* shoulders

The following exercises offer simple ways to strengthen some of the main muscle groups, which will help to stabilise your body and achieve an ideal posture. As with the 'stretch bank', these stretches may not be relevant until you have completed the 4 week programme, when you will be more aware of the long terms aims for your body and the areas that you would like to spend more time working on. They are there for you to work on at your leisure.

FISH TAIL – HALF

FISH TAIL – PADDLING

SEA BIRD

FISH TAIL – SIDEWAYS

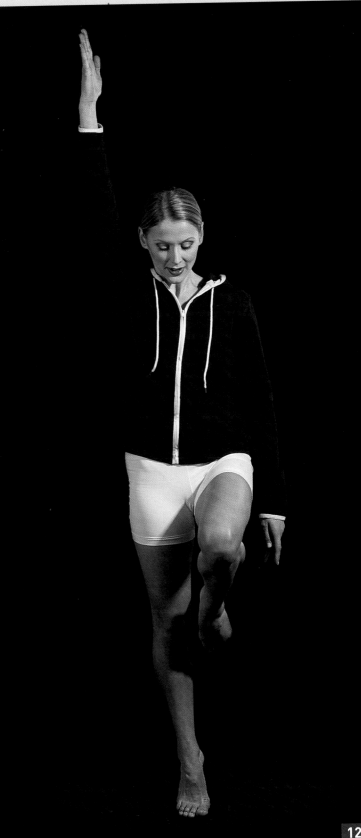

STRETCH BANKS

STRETCH BANK
Flamingo stretch **for the hands**

Muscle targets flexors and palms.

Main effects to shape the arms and wrists; to improve circulation throughout the whole arm area, including the shoulder and neck; to improve the flexibility of the hands.

Breathing Half Moon.

Position kneel on the floor, with your arms outstretched in front of you. Place your palms flat on the floor, with your fingers pointing back towards your body.

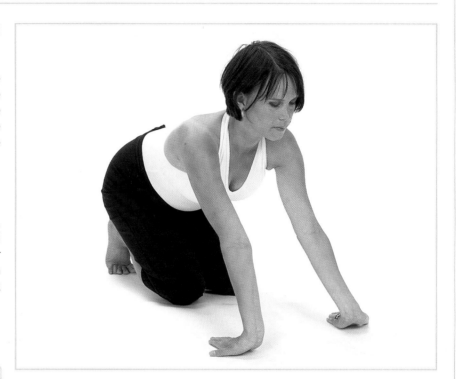

tip
If you find it hard to kneel for a long time, you can try this stretch against a wall. Stand with your palms flat on the wall and your fingers pointing down. You can deepen the stretch by pushing the heel of your hand into the wall and bending your knees.

Steps

* focus on the flexors and visualise a line of movement that travels up from the hand to the forearm.

* inhale.

* relax your hand and fingers.

* exhale, and gently start to push the heel of your hand into the floor.

* deepen the stretch by dropping your body weight back towards your heels, keeping your arms straight.

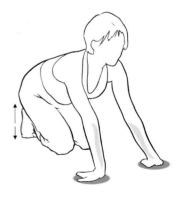

STRETCH BANK
Gibbon stretch

Muscle targets back and chest.

Main effects to lift the back; to shape the waistline; to pull the stomach in; to lift the chest; to reduce tension in the back; to alleviate tiredness.

Breathing Rising Sun.

Position stand facing a doorframe at arms length from it. Hook your hands onto the doorframe (with your right arm above the left), keeping your arms straight, at just above head height. Drop your shoulders and ribcage down, and drop your head slightly left and forward. Keep your feet next to each other, or put your right foot just over your left.

Steps

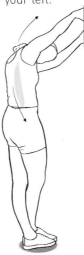

* focus on the right side of your upper back.

* breathe into your upper back and bend your knees slightly.

* exhale, PAUSE, create the stretch by straightening your legs, tilting your tailbone towards your navel, while keeping your head and upper back at the same level.

* create a deeper stretch by applying more body weight through the upper back by bending or extending your legs.

* repeat on the other side.

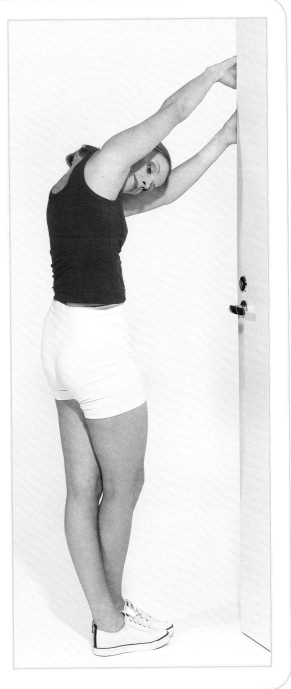

STRETCH BANKS

STRETCH BANK
Windsurfer stretch

Muscle targets back and chest.

Main effects to lift the back; to shape the waistline; to pull the stomach in; to lift the chest; to reduce tension in the back; to alleviate tiredness.

Breathing Half Moon.

Position assume a similar position as in the previous *Gibbon stretch*. Stand facing a doorframe at arm's length from it. Hook your hands onto the doorframe (right arm above the left), keeping your arms straight. This time place your arms lower, in line with you waist, and put your hands close together. Place your right leg over your left. Turn your right leg out from the hip socket and turn your tailbone towards your navel. Drop your shoulders and ribcage down. Relax your head, tilting it slightly left and forward, leading the curve of the spine.

Note Keep your shoulders stable. This is important in order to focus the stretch on your back. Engage your Abdominal Corset to focus your bodyweight towards your Centreline.

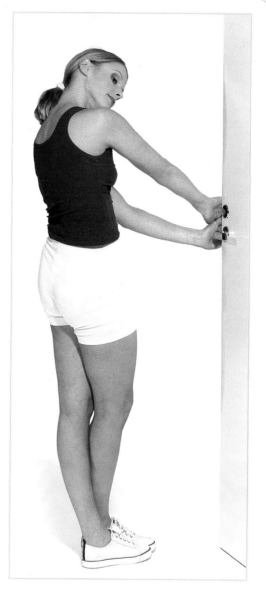

Steps

* focus on the right side of your upper back, all the way down to your lower back.

* inhale, allowing the pressure to open your back.

* exhale, and engage your abdominal corset to help you do this.

* apply weight through the muscles in your back. Slowly bend your right leg, working towards your Ground Point. Straighten your leg and tilt your tailbone towards your navel.

* repeat on the other side.

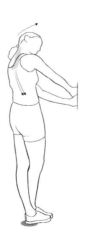

Note Control the stretch with your arms and legs, gradually applying more body weight through the upper back.

STABILISING BANK
Fish tail – half

Muscle targets inner thigh muscles.

Main effects to stabilise the pelvis.

Position lie on the floor on your right side, and support your head with your right arm. Turn your tailbone slightly towards your navel. Straighten your right leg and place the foot of your left leg on the floor in front of your right knee. Place your left hand on the floor.

Steps

* inhale using Half Moon breathing. Press your left hand into the floor; squeeze your sitting bones closer to each other, and lift your waistline off the floor.

* exhale, PAUSE, and lift the right leg about 10 cm off the floor. Use your Abdominal Corset to help support the leg.

* keep breathing deeply and slowly, and focus on the inner thigh muscles.

* repeat on the other side.

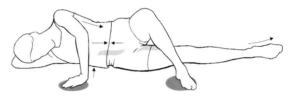

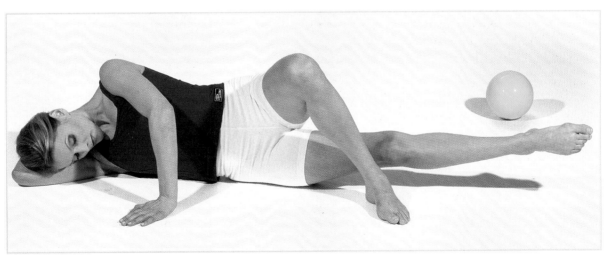

STABILISING BANK
Fish tail – paddling

Muscle targets lower buttocks, upper hamstrings.

Main effects to connect the leg muscles to the pelvis using the Abdominal Corset; to improve the position of the pelvis.

Position lie on your stomach and relax your forehead on the back of your hands. Lengthen your neck by bringing your chin towards your chest slightly, and straighten your legs.

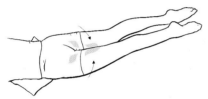

Steps

✸ inhale using Half Moon breathing.

✸ tilt your tailbone towards your Navel Point and lift your abdominal wall towards the front of your spine.

✸ lift both your Navel Point and your Diaphragm Point towards your spine.

✸ exhale, and press your pubic bone towards the floor (Ground Point); lift both legs about 5 cm off the floor.

✸ focus on your hamstrings running down the back of your legs.

✸ Keeping your pelvis still, begin to paddle with both of your legs as if you were swimming. Keep the pace quick, until each leg has paddled around 20 times.

✸ Keep your knees straight, but not locked.

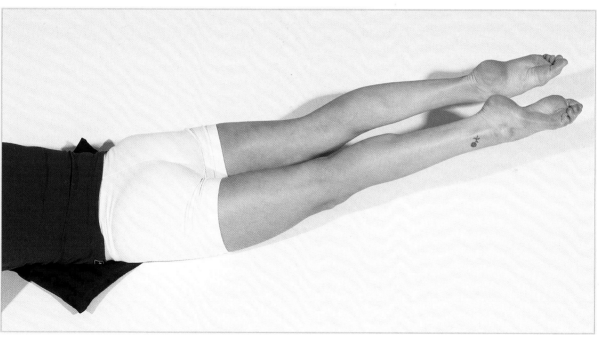

STABILISING BANK
Sea bird

Muscle targets upper arms, upper and lower back.

Main effects to connect the arms to the Abdominal Corset.

Breathing Half Moon.

Position lie on your stomach and relax your forehead onto the floor, or place a small pillow or cushion if it is more comfortable. Extend your arms along the length of your body, with your palms facing towards the ceiling. Press your forehead down, and keep the length in your neck.

Steps

❋ inhale.

❋ exhale, roll your shoulders back, and slowly lift your arms approximately 30 cm off the floor.

❋ slide your shoulder blades down your back towards your pelvis. Contract the muscles around your shoulder blades and your upper arms.

❋ inhale, and lower your arms so that they are approximately 5 cm off the floor.

❋ repeat this movement as many times as you feel comfortable.

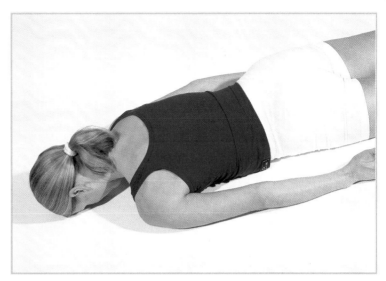

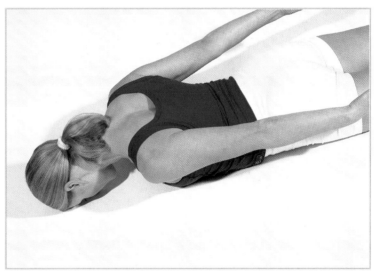

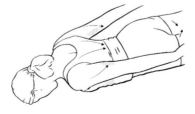

tip
Move your arms slowly enough to help you feel the muscles working. Imagine you are carrying something with your arms.

STABILISING BANK
Fish tail – sideways

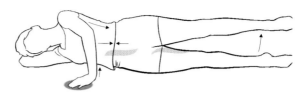

Muscle targets inner thighs; pelvic floor muscles.

Main effects to strengthen the deeper abdominals.

Position lie on your side, resting your head on your right arm. Place your left arm in front of your ribcage, bending your elbow and pointing your fingers up along your body. Straighten your legs and lift your waistline off the ground.

Steps

✳ inhale using Half Moon breathing.

✳ exhale, and working from your Abdominal Corset, lift both your legs off the floor.

✳ maintain this position, counting slowly to 6 as you inhale, and lowering your legs slowly as you exhale.

✳ repeat this move, this time lifting the upper leg slightly higher than the lower leg.

✳ return the upper leg back to the hip level, exhale and return both legs to the floor.

✳ repeat this exercise 3 times on each side.

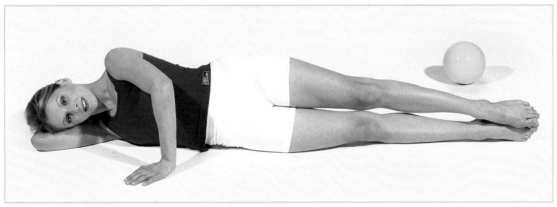

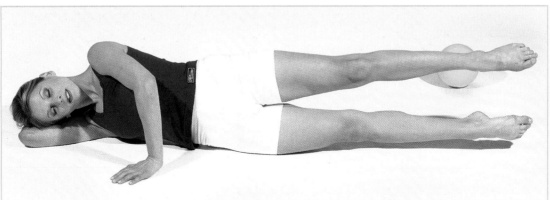

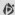

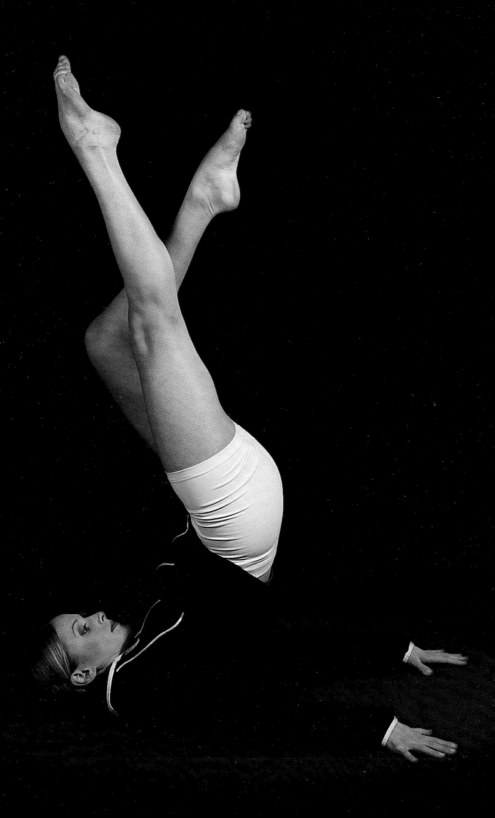

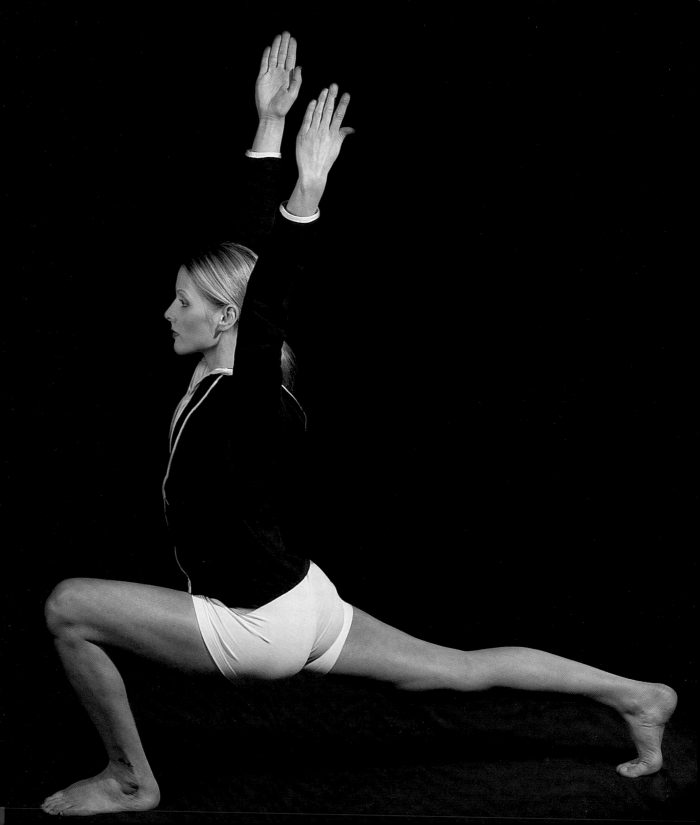

ELEMENTS AFFECTING YOUR RESULTS

NUTRITION

Your ability to strengthen and lengthen your muscles can be greatly influenced by the quality of your diet. Healthy muscles should be elastic, and the tissue covering your muscles should be slippery. The signs of a nutritional imbalance can manifest themselves as you stretch in terms of pain – not a 'bad' pain, but an uncomfortable type of pain that prevents your muscles from relaxing into stretches. Not eating well will increase the likelihood of suffering from aching muscles and joints, dry skin, fatigue and stiffness in the morning.

Eating well is another book in itself, but in general keep an eye on your daily vitamin and mineral intake; keep your sugar, fats and white bread intake down; and make sure that you drink plenty of water.

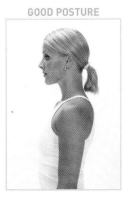

GOOD POSTURE

YOUR BODY TYPE

Knowing your body will help you become aware, not only of the possibilities, but also of your body's limitations.

YOUR POSTURAL CATEGORY

What category do you fall under? They can generally be divided into four:

1 good posture – where your shoulders are open and relaxed, your pelvis is held in a neutral position (not tilting backwards or forwards), and your head is aligned, leaving your neck open.

2 hunched posture – where your shoulders roll towards your chest, and your back curves forward too much.

3 sway back – where the back of your spine curves in too much.

4 military posture – where you back is too straight and rigid.

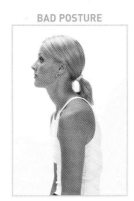

BAD POSTURE

You may be a mixture of more than one of these categories. However, recognising any problems with your posture will allow you to work towards correction.

YOUR MUSCLE TYPE

What type are you? Some people naturally build muscle tissue quite easily, while others struggle a little more.

Strong tissue

Sprinters usually fall into this category. Muscles are stronger and get big easily. They can work against very heavy resistance, but grow tired quickly.

Soft tissue

Long distance runners usually fall into this category. They tends to have leaner and thinner body types and find it easy to stretch.

Between the two

The third category is a mixed one, as many people fall between the two. This can provide them with a good readiness for many sports that demand different skills and capacities. For example, a football match lasts for 90 minutes, requiring stamina, but players will also be required to make lots of short quick sprints, requiring bursts of power. People in this category are often suited to mixed physical activity.

MUSCLE BALANCE

Our bodies are not symmetrical; they differ in bone structure, shape, size, length and placement on each side. During your programme you will become aware of the varying degrees of muscle shortness within your body.

Aim to lengthen the shorter muscles more intensively. For example, if you find that your pectoral muscles are shorter on the right side of your chest than they are on the left, spend more time working on the right side in order to balance yourself out. In general, if you feel that your muscles are fairly well balanced, then you should work on both sides of your body equally.

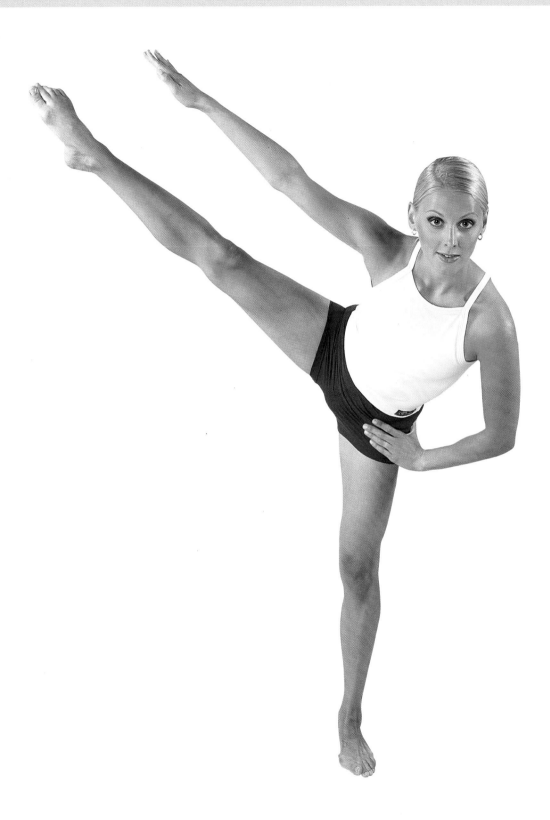

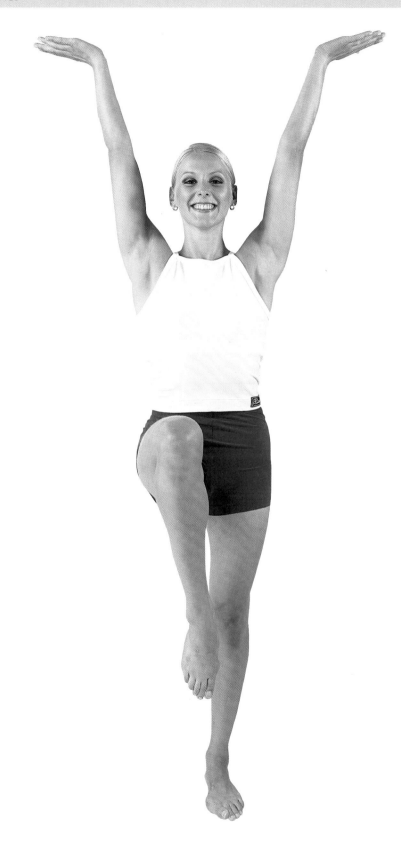

HOW TO MEASURE THE RESULTS

At the end of the 4 week programme you should be able to see and feel improvements in your posture, body shape and well-being. It is important that you are able to measure the improvement based on your own observations.

Now it's time to answer the second questionnaire, which is similar to the one that you completed at the start of the programme. Before you do, read through this section and think about your progress.

YOUR FIRST IMPRESSIONS

* do you have increased flexibility, allowing your body to maintain a better posture?
* do you feel that you have improved your overall well-being?
* do your everyday movements feel more free and easy?
* have the lines and silhouette of your body improved?

HOW DO YOU FEEL?

* can you make connections between the different muscles of your body, for example, do you feel your abdominal area when you move?
* what part of your body do you now use to initiate your movements?
* are you more aware of your body weight when you are lying down?

* can you visualise, or feel, the Centreline of your body when you are moving and stretching?
* are you able to PAUSE at the end of exhalation, allowing your breathing technique to help you stretch?
* are you able to work with your Stabilising Points (Diaphragm, Navel and Throat Points)?
* can you isolate the main muscle groups in your mind?
* are you able to create opposite forces within your body to help with the effectiveness of the stretch?
* can you feel the individual muscle stretching and elongating?

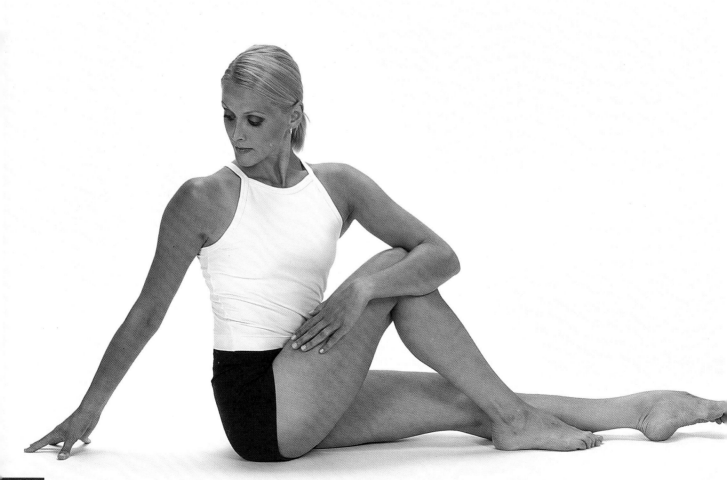

YOUR HEALTH & WELL-BEING

* do you feel less stressed and free from muscular tension?
* has your sleep improved?
* has your breathing technique and breathing capacity improved?
* do you feel stronger?
* are your muscles more supple and elastic?
* has your skin colour improved?
* has your circulation improved?
* do you feel more energetic?

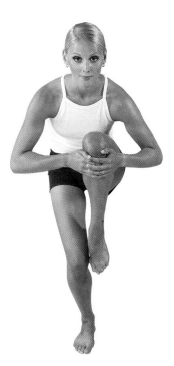

YOUR BODY ALIGNMENT

During the programme you have worked on elongating the tight, short muscles around your pelvis, as well as lifting your ribcage higher. Are you able to see how the shape of your body has become leaner, and how your posture has lifted?

Maintaining a good posture involves a subtle co-ordination of bones, ligaments, tendons, muscles and fascias to hold the body as a whole. To help you measure your improved posture, consider the following factors:

* how is the ribcage positioned in relation to the pelvis? Has you waist lengthened?

* are you aware of the support of your Abdominal Corset in the movements that you make, even when you are walking?

* has the position of your pelvis improved – does it naturally sit in a neutral position, rather than tilting?

* do you feel that the positioning of your shoulders has changed?

For the first time I can feel my shoulder blades moving as if they were heavier

**Minna,
Method Putksito client**

RESULTS
QUESTIONNAIRE

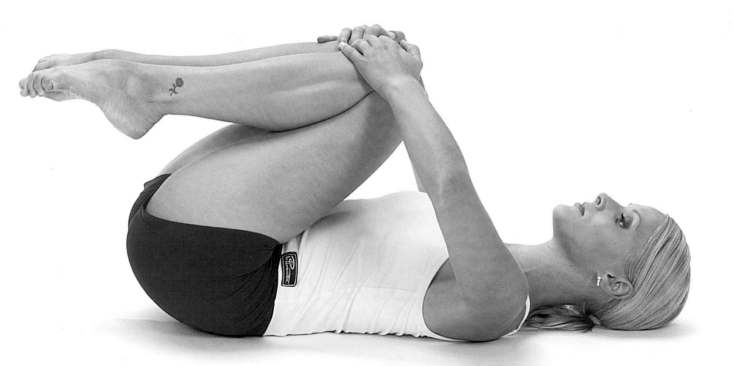

1 Have your achievements matched your original expectations of this programme? If not, how do they differ?

2 What improvements have you seen in your:

appearance?

performance?

3 How would you describe your body? (in three words)

4 How would you describe your posture? (in three words)

5 Rate your energy levels on a scale of 1–4
(1 = low, 4 = high).

| 1 | 2 | 3 | 4 |

6 Rate the quality of sleep you experience on a scale of 1–4. (1 = broken sleep, 4 = well-rested)

| 1 | 2 | 3 | 4 |

7 Rate the quality of your breathing on a scale of 1–4. (1 = shallow, inefficient breathing, 4 = deep, effective breathing)

| 1 | 2 | 3 | 4 |

8 Rate your range and ease of movement on a scale of 1-4. (1= difficult movement, 4 = full ease of movement)

| 1 | 2 | 3 | 4 |

9 Rate your muscle balance (do you feel shorter or tighter on one side?) on a scale of 1–4.
(1 = severe imbalance, 4 = perfect balance)

| 1 | 2 | 3 | 4 |

10 Do your muscles feel elastic or inelastic, on a scale of 1–4. (1 = inelastic, 4 = elastic)

| 1 | 2 | 3 | 4 |

11 Rate your flexibility on a scale of 1–4.
(1 = inflexible, 4 = flexible)

| 1 | 2 | 3 | 4 |

12 Now that you have finished your programme, have you been able to identify areas that have been particularly problematic, and may require more work?

13 Do you now feel able to trust your intuition and make choices more independently? Have you thought about how to create a longer-term stretching programme that will continue to benefit your body?

MOVING ON!

As you finish the programme and move back into your everyday life, think about your priorities. Perhaps one of the following options is important to you:

- to continue to improve your figure and lift your posture.
- to relax, recuperate, aid recovery from stress and increase your energy levels.
- to improve your stretching technique, increase your knowledge of your body and improve your concentration skills.

Now is the time to follow you own targets.

MAINTAINING THE RESULTS

Maintenance is *much easier* than the process of reaching your target – however the programme will not remain successful unless it is maintained.

To maintain your new muscle length, revert your emphasis from deep stretching to normal stretching; once or twice a week. If you prefer, you could continue to follow the deep stretching programme – for example once a week. You can even mix the two – following a normal stretching programme, but having a deep stretch 'top-up' whenever you feel your body needs it!

Although the results from following a regular deep stretching programme will be even more rewarding, there may be times in your life when you prefer to work with a less intensive programme. This is fine, and even a normal stretching session once a week is better than no stretching at all. You may even be able to incorporate some of the stretches into your everyday life.